Microskin Grafting for Vitiligo

Devendra K Gupta

Microskin Grafting for Vitiligo

Springer

Devendra K Gupta
Devendra Hospital and Yuva
Cosmetic Clinic
Bareilly, U.P. India

ISBN: 978-1-4471-6879-9 ISBN: 978-1-84882-605-2 (eBook)
DOI: 10.1007/978-1-84882-605-2
Springer Dordrecht Heidelberg London New York

Softcover re-print of the Hardcover 1st edition 2009

Printed on acid-free paper.

Springer is part of Springer Science+Business Media (www.springer.com)

Preface

This book has been written to assist not only postgraduate students, but also interested dermatologists, general practitioners, and surgeons.

During the last two decades, various surgical therapies have been used in the treatment of stable refractory vitiligo, but none of them became very popular because of their intrinsic drawbacks, and thus could not be adopted as a standard procedure. There has always been a need for a technique that gives best results without complications.

The commonly used surgical procedures for the treatment of vitiligo have been narrated in short and their characteristic drawbacks have been pointed out. The cellular graft technique is costly, requires a good laboratory and infrastructure, and except for being able to cover a wider vitiliginous area, the ultimate results are no better than tissue grafting technique. I used the small skin particles prepared from ultra thin or thin split thickness skin graft, the so called "microskin graft," in the treatment of vitiligo effectively with good expansion ratio, i.e., small donor skin to treat big vitiliginous area. This procedure covers the benefit of cellular and tissue graft, but without their inherent drawbacks.

The microskin graft technique has been illustrated with minimum necessary text to explain the steps. This technique is very simple to learn and execute. It is extremely cost effective and can treat very large area up to 1,500 cm^2 in an operative session. Even budding surgical specialists or dermatologists can start using this technique without any difficulty.

The only thing to be kept in mind before embarking surgical procedure is the *stability* of the vitiligo disease process.

Bareilly, India | Devendra K. Gupta

Acknowledgements

I am grateful to all my operation theatre staff who contributed to the refinement of the techniques and the quality of photographs.

I have taken away the time that was really destined for my wife Mrs. Vandana Devendra and children Shruti Devendra and Samarth Devendra for the preparation of this book. Their continuous moral support and encouragement made me complete this work on time. There are no words to express my gratitude to them.

I will never forget the time-to-time help extended to me by Dr. V. K. Chawla and Dr. Pawan kumar Agrawal for the preparation of this book. I also express thanks to Mr. Grant Weston, Cate Rogers, Padmaja Sudhakher and other staff at Springer for their outstanding help.

Contents

Abbreviations

AOR	(Appearance Of Repigmentation)
CEG	(Cultured Epithelial Grafts)
CM	(Cultured "pure" Melanocytes)
DA	(Donor Area)
EMLA	(Eutectic Mixture of Local Anesthetics)
FTSG	(Full Thickness Skin Graft)
FTSG-MPG	(Full Thickness Skin Graft-Mini Punch Graft) – 1–1.2 mm
HFG	(Hair Follicular Graft)
MPG	(Mini Punch Graft)
MSGs	(MicroSkin Grafts)
MSG	(MicroSkin graft)
8-MOP	(8-MethOxy-Psoralen)
MPS	(Maximum Pigment Spread)
MBG	(Micro Blister Graft)
MBEHQ	(MonoBenzyl Ether of HydroQuinone)
MED	(Minimal Erythematous Dose)
NCES	(Non-Cultured Epidermal cell Suspension)
OMP	(Oral Mini Pulse therapy)
OP	(Operative)
PABA	(Para-AminoBenzoic Acid)
PUVA	(Psoralen plus UltraViolet-A therapy)
PUVASOL	(Psoralen plus UltraViolet-A of SOLar origin)
RA	(Recipient Area)
SSG	(Split-Skin Grafting)
STSG	(Split Thickness Skin Graft)
SPs	(Skin Particles)
STSG-UT	(Split Thickness Skin Graft-Ultra Thin) = (0.08–0.15 mm)
STSG-T	(Split Thickness Skin Graft-Thin) = (0.2–0.3 mm)
STSG-M	(Split Thickness Skin Graft-Medium thickness) = (0.30–0.45 mm)
STSG-THK	(Split Thickness Skin Graft-Thick) = (0.45–0.75 mm)
STSG-BE	(Split Thickness Skin Graft – Blister Epidermal/Suction blister epidermal graft)
TBSA	(Total Body Surface Area)
TMP	(TriMethyl Psoralen)

Part I

Surgical Management

1 Surgical Therapies

1.1 Introduction

Vitiligo is a relatively common pigmentary disorder (affecting nearly 1–2% of population) of great socio-medical importance. Depigmentation of the skin with the loss of melanocytes on histology characterizes this disorder. It is defined as a circumscribed, acquired, idiopathic, progressive, hypomelanosis of skin and hair, often familial and characterized by total absence of melanocytes microscopically. This definition excludes postinflammatory, chemically induced depigmentation, and those which are associated with melanoma, secondary to various dermatoses and after burns. A range of clinical phenotypes lead to varying degrees of morbidity. The cause of vitiligo remains unknown, although an autoimmune pathogenesis seems most likely. Treatment also remains difficult. A number of new therapies show significant potential.

Vitiligo presents as sharply demarcated depigmented macules, that can appear anywhere on the skin. There is a predilection for orifices – eyes, nostrils, mouth, nipples, umbilicus, and genitalia.[1]The natural history of the disorder is either that it spreads quite quickly (over months) and then is stable, or it relentlessly spreads over the body with time (over years). Sites of trauma (koebnerization), such as the elbows, may develop vitiligo.[1] Twenty-three to twenty-six percent of patients are children under the age of twelve.[2–4] It is the most commonly acquired hypomelanosis.[5]

The typical Vitiligo macules have a well defined light tan border and are chalky or snow white (trichrome Vitiligo),[6] the fourth color being the dark brown macules of repigmentation which are usually perifollicular (quadrichrome vitiligo)[7]. Sometimes there may also be a hyperpigmented border or a red halo (inflammatory vitiligo).

Segmental Vitiligo presents in dermatomal, multi-dermatomal, quasidermatomal forms which are arranged unilaterally. Most patients do not develop lesions elsewhere. Vitiligo of distal digits and the lips produces the lip-tip syndrome. Bilateral lesions may be symmetrical or asymmetrical. Palms and soles are commonly involved. Mucosal depigmentation, including gingiva, genitalia, lips and nipples, leukotrichia – depigmented hair is common in Vitiligo patches.

Vitiligo can be extremely disfiguring, leading to significant patient morbidity. A number of different studies have been carried out to measure the quality of life for patients with vitiligo. Low self-esteem, poor body image and poor quality of life has been found in patients with vitiligo, including significant psychiatric morbidity (up to 25% in one study).[8]

Vitiligo or Leukoderma as it is more familiarly known in many parts of the world has gained importance principally because of the serious social stigma especially in the dark skinned people. It can be devastating to their self esteem because the sufferer may face problems related to matrimonial alliance or even in getting employment. It is very common in the countries like Pakistan, India and Bangladesh.

1.2 Course and Prognosis

Vitiligo is a chronic disease process. The course is highly variable but rapid onset followed by a period of stability or slow progress is most characteristic. Up to 30% may report some spontaneous repigmentation particularly in sun-exposed areas. Rapidly progressive or "galloping" Vitiligo may lead to extensive depigmentation.

D. K. Gupta, *Microskin Grafting for Vitiligo*,
DOI: 10.1007/978-1-84882-605-2_1, © Springer Science + Business Media B.V. 2009

Vitiligo zosteriformis/segmental, however, is the most stable form and may show a better prognosis.[9,10] Segmental Vitiligo is a special subset which usually develops precipitously in a region, which does not usually extend beyond quasidermatomal region, and is very stable, once present.

A few of the cases may once again start progressing at a rapid pace after a period of dormancy. Such an occurrence is not uncommon in nonsegmental vitiligo types namely vitiligo vulgaris, acrofacialis and areata. In addition, several other factors may assist in evaluating its prognosis, (a) the younger the patient, the shorter the duration, the better is the prognosis, (b) the lesions located on the fleshy regions of the body may show better chance of recovery in contrast to that on bony/friction points and (c) the presence of leukotrichia or lesions on mucous membranes or mucocutaneous junctions may account for a poor prognosis.[10]

Another important aspect in the management of vitiligo is to identify the prognostic factors in each patient as this would be essential to decide on the end point of any modality of therapy. In my experience, a poor prognostic factor includes history of progression, family history of vitiligo, widespread disease, nonsegmental vitiligo, acrofacial vitiligo. I would also advise that all patients of vitiligo should be given sunscreens, antioxidants and options regarding cosmetic camouflage. Finally, the management of vitiligo would not be complete without good counseling, motivation and psychological support to the patient.

1.3 Surgical Therapies

The most frequently used treatment for vitiligo is PUVA (psoralen plus ultraviolet A) and/or topical or systemic steroids.[11] It has been reported that these standard treatments result in limited success rates (about 60% of patients achieve more than 25% repigmentation).These refractory and stable vitiligo can be subjected to various surgical therapies.

All the surgical therapies used in vitiligo are categorized into either the tissue grafts or the cellular grafts. The tissue grafts are simple ones and used to give good repigmentary results without the need of hi-tech laboratory and infrastructure, but the disadvantage is that, only limited vitiliginous area can be treated at a time. The cellular grafts are the latest one to be used in vitiligo and include both cultured and non cultured melanocytes and promise to cover wide vitiliginous area in one operative session with limited donor site. The tissue grafts includes split thickness skin grafts, mini punch grafts, hair follicle grafts and suction blister epidermal grafts. These current surgical treatments for stable refractory vitiligo are overviewed.

1.4 Split Thickness Skin Sheet Grafting

This method removes the epidermis and superficial papillary dermis of vitiligo depigmented areas by dermabrasion, and replaces it with very thin dermo-epidermal grafts harvested from normally pigmented donor skin with a dermatome.[12] Although the method is simple, the motor-driven diamond fraise or wire brush used for dermabrasion at recipient sites sometimes leaves a hypertrophic scar if dermabrasion is done deeply and harvesting excessively thick grafts can also result in hypopigmentation or slight scarring at donor sites. Apart from this there is characteristic recipient area deformities like achromic fissuring, stuck-on appearance, perigraft hypopigmented halo and rolled up peripheral margin.

1.5 Minipunch Grafting

This method consists of harvesting small (1.0–1.2 mm) punches of graft skin from donor sites and transferring these minigrafts to the vitiligo recipient sites, separated 3–4 mm from each other.[13–15] Repigmentation occurs within several months by coalescence of pigmentation arising from the small grafted islands, but sunlight exposure for 10–15 min daily or ultraviolet A (UVA) irradiation may assist in repigmentation. Usually 4–5 mm of centrifugal pigmentation occurs around each recipient site, corresponding to approximately 20–25 times its original size. This procedure is excellent for segmental vitiligo, but sometimes a cobblestone appearance or scarring may result at the recipient site and donor site, which can be more noticeable with minigrafts larger than 1.2 mm.

1.6 Suction Blisters Epidermal Grafting

This method is performed in two stages.[16,17] First, recipient sites are ablated by freezing with liquid nitrogen or blister induced by PUVA, which is performed 2 days prior to grafting. Secondly, blisters are formed at donor sites via a suction apparatus at –200 to –300 mmHg for 2–3 hours. This method can also be done in one stage by dermabrading the recipient sites by diamond fraise and raising blisters from donor site simultaneously in one operative session. After the roof of the blister is removed from the donor sites, the donor epidermis is placed on top of the dermabraded skin at the recipient sites with correct orientation. Repigmentation occurs by proliferation of melanocytes and spreading of pigment from grafts. The advantages of this procedure are, a low incidence of scarring and the possibility of reusing the donor site for future treatments, but it takes 2–3 hours to make the suction blisters and it is not easy to treat extensive vitiliginous areas in one operative session. There are more chances of hyperpigmentation at both donor and recipient areas particularly in initial months of procedure.

1.7 Transplantation of Cultured or Noncultured Melanocytes

A new era has begun in surgical therapy with the development of transplantation techniques with cultured or noncultured melanocytes. This procedure allows the treatment of larger areas in shorter periods. Lerner and colleagues[18] successfully treated a patient of piebaldism by injecting cultured melanocytes into small blisters raised on areas devoid of pigment. Olsson and Juhlin[19,20] using cultured melanocytes have reported repigmentation of vitiligo in 10 and 100 patients, respectively. Further evolution has led to noncultured epidermal cell transplantation. Olsson and Juhlin[21] have reported excellent results using epidermal cell transplantation on 26 patients in their outpatient clinic. Gauthier and Surleve-Bazeille[22] have described grafting with noncultured melanocytes and keratinocytes. They injected cell suspension into blisters produced with liquid nitrogen. The scalp was chosen as the donor area. However, it is a 2-day procedure and limits treatment to only a very small area in one operative session. Van Geel and colleagues[23] conducted a pilot study of only four patients with noncultured melanocytes and keratinocytes grafted on superficially laser dermabraded vitiligo lesions.

These transplanting techniques have the theoretical advantage of potentially treating large areas using cells harvested from a small piece of donor skin by expanding the culture in vitro. But its major disadvantage lies in the complexities and cost of the culture. Also, more knowledge of the biology and safety of in vitro cultured cells is necessary before cultured cells are used in daily practice.

In order to overcome the deficiencies of these current treatments for stable refractory vitiligo, I have developed a new method to treat vitiligo which used mechanical superficial dermabrasion and microskin grafting. Patients with stable segmental or generalized vitiligo on their body sites can be treated using this method. Each operation has been very successful, and excellent repigmentation is observed at all grafting sites without producing any scar on donor and recipient sites. Strict superficial dermabrasion with a diamond fraise leaves no scar on recipient areas. Microskin grafting can cover a wider area (donor to recipient area ratio up to 1:15) from a smaller donor site compared with the sheet skin grafting technique. PUVA treatment may then be given to promote the spreading of pigmentation particularly in generalized type of vitiligo but not in segmental vitiligo.

Thus, if topical or systemic steroids or PUVA treatment fail to repigment vitiligo vulgaris, surgical alternatives exist, which include autografting, suction blisters grafting, split thickness skin sheet grafting, mini punch grafting and transplantation of cultured or non cultured melanocytes, and the last but not the least, the microskin grafting, a most successful and excellent repigmentation procedure even in generalized stable vitiligo.

References

1. Schwartz RA, Janniger CK. Vitiligo. *Cutis*. 1997;60: 239–244.
2. Hann SK, Chang JH, Lee HS, Kim SM. The classification of segmental vitiligo on the face. *Yonsei Med J*. 2000;41: 209–212.
3. Halder RM, Grimes PE, Cowan CA, Enterline JA, Chakrabarti SG, Kenney JA. Childhood vitiligo. *J Am Acad Dermatol*. 1987;16:948–954.
4. Jaisankar TJ, Baruah MC, Garg BR. Vitiligo in children. *Int J Dermatol*. 1992;31(9):621–623.

5. Taieb A. Intrinsic and extrinsic pathomechanisms in vitiligo. *Pigment Cell Res*. 2000;13:41–47.
6. Dupre A, Christol B. Cockade - like vitiligo and linear vitiligo a variant of Fitzpatrick's trichrome vitiligo. *Arch Dermatol Res*. 1978;262:197–203.
7. Behl PN, Aggarwal A, Srivastava G. Vitiligo. In: Behl PN, Srivastava G, eds. *Practice of Dermatology*. 9th ed. New Delhi: CBS Publishers; 2003:238–241.
8. Mattoo SK, Handa S, Kaur I, Gupta N, Malhotra R. Psychiatric morbidity in vitiligo: prevalence and correlates in India. *J Eur Acad Dermatol Venereol*. 2002;16: 573–578.
9. Sehgal VN, Rege VL, Mascarenhas F, Kharangate VN. Clinical pattern of vitiligo amongst Indians. *J Dermatol Tokyo*. 1976;3:49–53.
10. Michaelsson G. Vitiligo with raised borders. Report of two cases. *Acta Derm Venereol*. 1968;48:158–161.
11. Drake LA, Dinehart SM, Farmer ER, et al. Guideline of care for vitiligo. *J Am Acad Dermatol*. 1996;35:620–626.
12. Kahn AM, Cohen MJ. Vitiligo: treatment by dermabrasion and epithelial sheet grafting. *J Am Acad Dermatol*. 1995; 33:646–648.
13. Falabella R. Treatment of localized vitiligo by autologous minigraft-ing. *Arch Dermatol*. 1988;124:1649–1655.
14. Boersma BR, Westerhof W, Bos JD. Repigmentation in vitiligo vulgaris by autologous minigrafting: results in nineteen patients. *J Am Acad Dermatol*. 1995;33:990–995.
15. Malakar S, Dhar S. Treatment of stable and recalcitrant vitiligo by autologous miniature punch grafting: a prospective study of 1000 patients. *Dermatology*. 198:1999;133–139.
16. Koga M. Epidermal grafting using the tops of suction blisters in the treatment of vitiligo. *Arch Dermatol*. 1988;124: 1656–1658.
17. Hann SK, Im S, Bong HW, Park YK. Treatment of stable vitiligo with autologous epidermal grafting and PUVA. *J Am Acad Dermatol*. 1995;32:943–9485.
18. Lerner AB, Halaban R, Klaus SN, Mollemann GE. Transplantation of human melanocytes. *J Invest Dermatol*. 1987;89:219–224.
19. Olsson MJ, Juhlin L. Repigmentation of vitiligo by transplantation of cultured autologous melanocytes. *Acta Dermatol Venereol (Stock)*. 1993;73:49–51.
20. Olsson MJ, Juhlin L. Transplantation of melanocytes in vitiligo. *Br J Dermatol*. 1995;132:587–591.
21. Olsson MJ, Juhlin L. Leucoderma treated by transplantation of basal cell layer enriched suspension. *Br J Dermatol*. 1998;138:644–648.
22. Gauthier Y, Surleve-Bazeille J. Autologous grafting with non cultured malanocytes: a simplified method for treatment of depigmented lesions. *J Am Acad Dermatol*. 1992;26:191–194.
23. Van Geel N, Ongeane K, De Mil M, et al. Modified technique of autologous non-cultured epidermal cell transplantation for repigmenting vitiligo: a pilot study. *Dermatol Surg*. 2001;27:873–876.

Concept of the Stability of Vitiligo

2

Although the treatment of vitiligo has reasonably improved in the last decade, the results are still not satisfying for many patients. This is probably due to the fact that the etiopathogenesis is unknown. Several treatment modalities, such as PUVA, UVB and local corticosteroids are currently used in the treatment of active vitiligo. However, these treatments usually induce incomplete repigmentation. Surgical methods[1] intended to repigment vitiligo are interesting therapeutic option if patients have stable disease. Before planning surgical therapies, stability of vitiligo must be confirmed. Following points should be kept in mind:

1. Grafting in vitiligo should be resorted to, when the disease is stable and has been refractory to medical line of treatment. Such cases are called as stable vitiligo (quiescent vitiligo).
2. This indicates that functioning melanocytes are no more available in the refractory patches of vitiligo.
3. If these patches are repopulated with autologous functioning melanocytes, then the vitiligo patches will repigment again.

Patients are recruited for surgical procedures based on certain clinical criteria including[1–3]

- Disease, which is stable for at least 1 year.
- Failure of appropriate and adequate medical therapy.
- Localized vitiligo (Focal, segmental, mucosal).

Stability of the disease is the most important factor, which must be ensured before undertaking surgical procedures, and it is preferable to put a graft before proceeding with the full procedure. Surgical procedures can be followed with application of topical PUVASOL once the acute edema of the procedure has subsided to enhance spread of the transplanted functioning melanocytes.

2.1 Stability

Surgery is indicated for all types of stable vitiligo including segmental, generalized and acrofacial types that do not respond to medical treatment. The outcome of the surgery is good in stable lesions, whereas, unstable lesions respond poorly. Thus, the stability status of vitiligo is the single, most important prerequisite in case selection. However, despite many studies, there is no consensus regarding the minimum required period of stability. Stability has been defined by different authors as a period varying from 4 months to 3 years during which the existing lesions should not have enlarged, no new lesions should have appeared, and there should be no koebnerization[2–6].Most authors have suggested that vitiligo can be classified as being stable when there is no progression of old lesions and/or development of new lesions during the past 1 year. It is best to confirm the stability of the disease in doubtful cases by doing trial test grafting in a small vitiliginous area 1.5–2 months before undertaking surgery of the entire lesion.[7,8]

A set of objective criteria-the vitiligo disease activity score (VIDA), was suggested by Njoo et al[6,9] in 1999 to follow the progress of the patient. It is a 6-point scale on which the activity of the disease is evaluated by the appearance of new vitiligo lesions or the enlargement of preexisting lesions gauged during a period ranging from <6 weeks to 1 year (Table 2.1). It is recommended that surgery for vitiligo should be performed only in patients with VIDA scores of −1 or 0.

D. K. Gupta, *Microskin Grafting for Vitiligo*,
DOI: 10.1007/978-1-84882-605-2_2, © Springer Science + Business Media B.V. 2009

Table 2.1 VIDA 6-point score[6,9]

Disease activity	VIDA score
Active in past 6 weeks	+4
Active in past 3 months	+3
Active in past 6 months	+2
Active in past 1 year	+1
Stable for at least 1 year	0
Stable for at least 1 year and spontaneous repigmentation	−1

2.2 Minigraft Test[7,8]

Four to six minigrafts of 1.0–1.2 mm were implanted within lesions of patients with unilateral (localized) and bilateral (generalized) vitiligo (Figs. 2.1–2.3). Pigment spread was assessed 3 months later. The unilateral vitiligo patients (95%) had a positive test result in comparison with patients (48%) with bilateral vitiligo ($p = 0.002$). The minigrafting test is a reliable tool to identify patients with stable vitiligo who may respond to melanocyte transplantation. Unilateral (localized) vitiligo is the best indication for surgical repigmentation. Patients were selected for grafting when spread of pigment was observed within 3 months. In all patients with a positive Koebner phenomenon

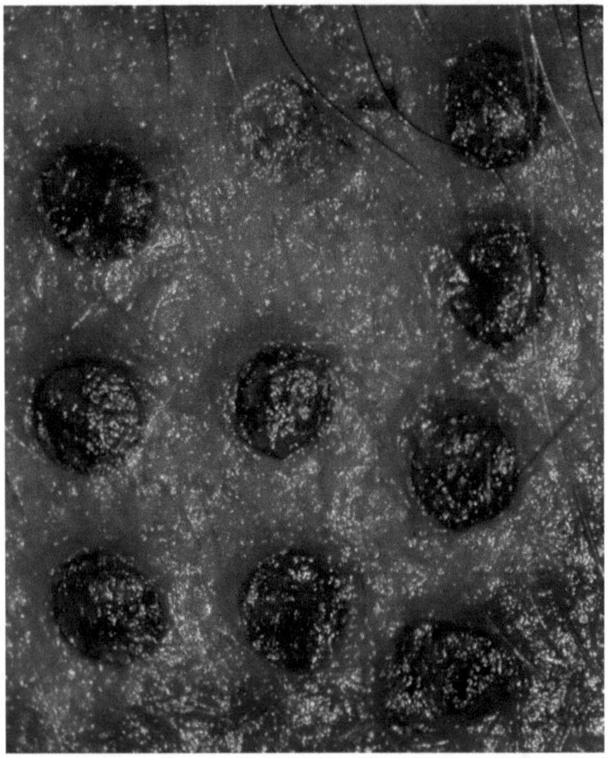

Fig. 2.2 Appearance of repigmentation (AOR) from MPGs on 11th day

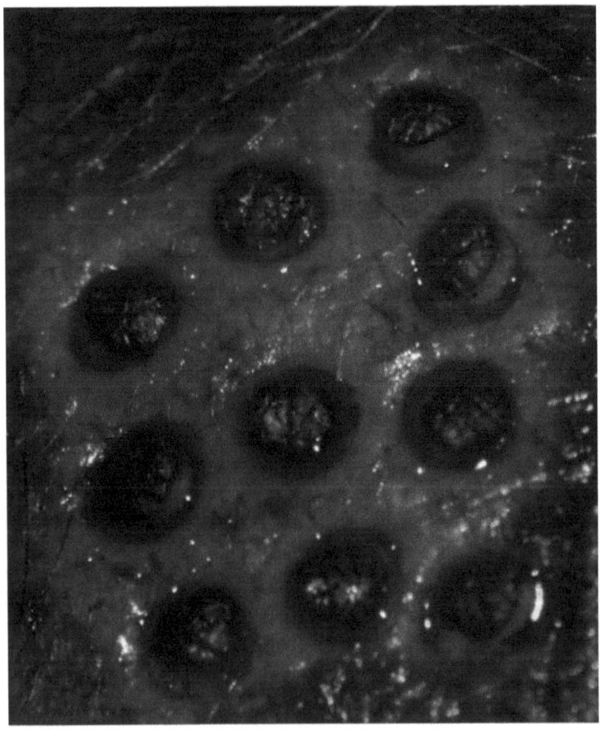

Fig. 2.1 1.2 mm mini punch grafts (MPGs) transplanted within lesion

Fig. 2.3 Pigmentation completed in 50 days

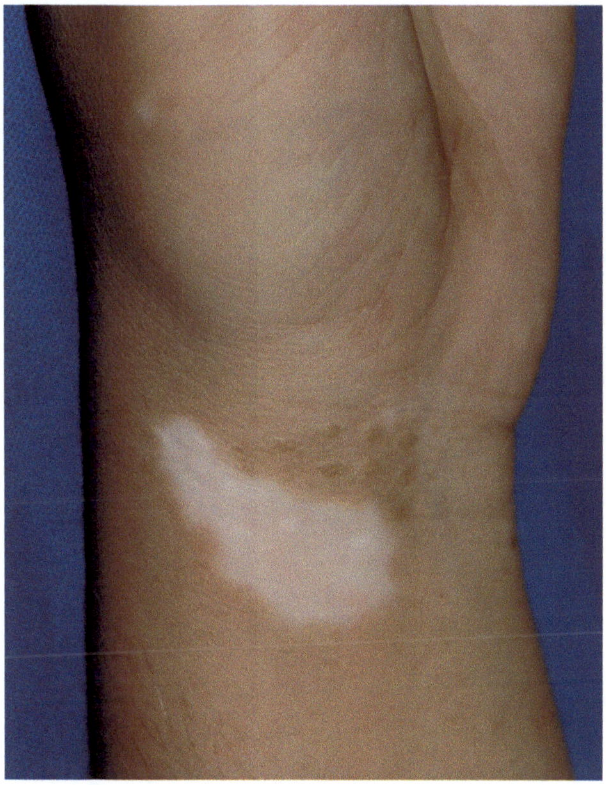

Fig. 2.4 In a positive Koebner phenomenon depigmentation of the minigrafts developed

depigmentation of the minigrafts developed (Fig. 2.4). Selected patients with stable and refractory vitiligo may consider melanocyte transplantation as a therapeutic alternative.

I believe that stationary or decreasing lesions, and non appearance of new lesions for at least 1 year is supposed to be a better criteria for selection of patient for surgery rather than minigraft test itself.

References

1. Van Geel N, Ongenae K, Naeyaert JM. Surgical techniques for vitiligo: a review. *Dermatology*. 2001;202(2):162–166.
2. Savant SS. Autologous miniature punch skin grafting in stable vitiligo. *Indian J Dermatol Venereol Leprol*. 1992;58:310–314.
3. Boersma BR, Westerhof W, Bos JD. Repigmentation in vitiligo vulgaris by autologous minigrafting: results in nineteen patients. *J Am Acad Dermatol*. 1995;33:990–995.
4. Njoo MD, Westerhof W, Bos JD, Bossuyt MM. A systematic review of autologous transplantation methods in vitiligo. *Arch Dermatol*. 1998;134:1543–1545.
5. Guerra L, Capurro S, Melchi F. Treatment of "stable" vitiligo by timed surgery and transplantation of cultured epidermal autografts. *Arch Dermatol*. 2000;136:1380–1389.
6. Parsad D, Gupta S. Standard guidelines of care for vitiligo surgery. *Indian J Dermatol Venereol Leprol*. 2008;74:37–45.
7. Falabella R, Arrunategui A, Barona MI, Alzate A. The minigrafting test for vitiligo: detection of stable lesions for melanocytes transplantation. *J Am Acad Dermatol*. 1995;32: 228–232.
8. Westerhof W, Boersma BR. The minigrafting test for vitiligo: detection of stable lesions for melanocytes transplantation. *J Am Acad Dermatol*. 1995;33:1061–1062.
9. Njoo MD, Das PK, Bos JD, Westerhof W. Association of the Kobner phenomenon with disease activity and therapeutic responsiveness in vitiligo vulgaris. *Arch Dermatol*. 1999;135: 407–413.

Classification of Surgical Treatment Modalities

3

In vitiligo, there is a partial or total destruction of melanocytes, initially only of the epidermis, and later even of the hair follicle, which acts as a reservoir for providing melanocytes during repigmentation.[1] Hence, in patients with vitiligo, the existing melanocytes need to be activated. While medical therapies are the primary treatment, there are some patients refractory to medical treatment. In such patients, surgical therapies can be used either alone or in conjunction with medical therapy to achieve repigmentation, provided the disease is stable.

Three types of surgical techniques are available: excision with primary closure, tissue grafts and cellular grafts, with in between autologous cultured epithelial grafts for the repopulation of depleted melanocytes in vitiligo. With tissue grafts, only a limited surface area can be treated, but with good results in a majority of cases. Starting from autologous cellular suspensions, epithelial grafts of various compositions can be cultured in vitro. The cellular grafts can be used for larger areas.

For convenience, the tissue grafts and cellular grafts can be classified as follows:

3.1 Classification of Tissue Grafts[2]

Tissue grafts (Fig. 3.1):

- Split-thickness skin graft (STSG)
- Full thickness skin graft (FTSG)

3.1.1 Split-Thickness Skin Grafts (STSG) (Fig. 3.1)

In free split thickness skin sheet graft, the epidermis or the epidermis and varying thickness of dermis are cut during harvesting of graft (Detail in Chapter 5 & 6).

- Split-thickness skin graft-blister epidermis (STSG-BE)
- Split-thickness skin graft-ultra-thin (STSG-UT)
- Split-thickness skin graft-thin (STSG-T)
- Split-thickness skin graft-medium (STSG-M)
- Split-thickness skin graft-thick (STSG-THK)

3.1.2 Full Thickness Skin Graft (FTSG) (Fig. 3.1)

In FTSG, the epidermis and full thickness of dermis are cut during graft harvesting. FTSG can be cut as small disc of epidermis along with full dermis, so called MPG, for transplantation for repigmentory surgery of vitiligo. HFG is like MPG but it contain a single hair follicle and a thin sleeve of epidermis and full dermis. (Detail in Chapter 7).

D. K. Gupta, *Microskin Grafting for Vitiligo*,
DOI: 10.1007/978-1-84882-605-2_3, © Springer Science + Business Media B.V. 2009

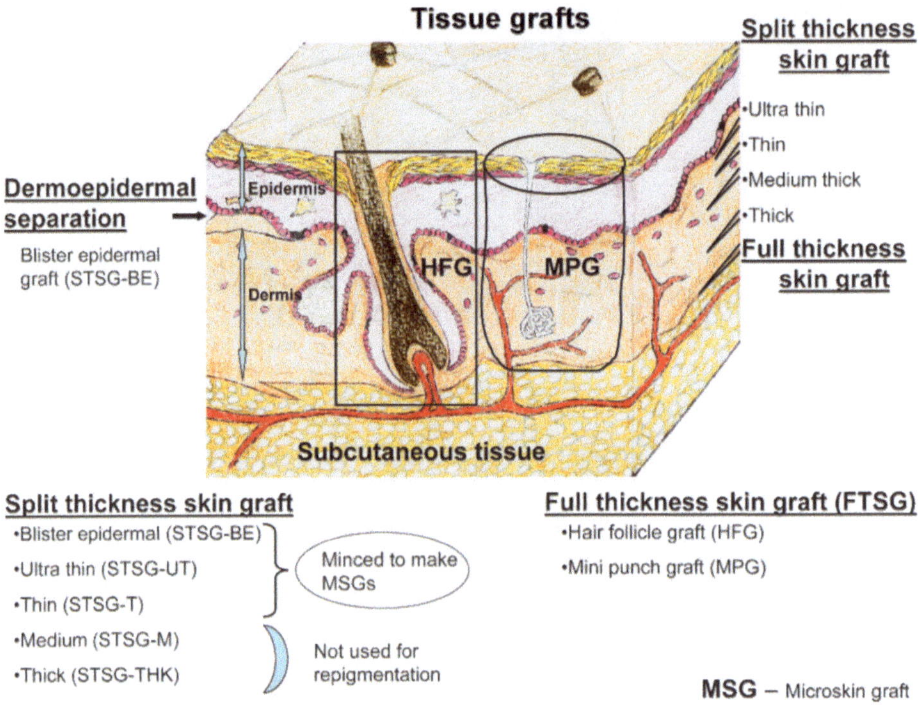

Fig. 3.1 Classification of tissue grafts used for repigmentation surgery. The thickness of the various types of free skin grafts, showing the constituent of each

- Mini-punch graft (MPG)
- Hair follicular graft (HFG)

3.2 Classification of Cellular Grafts

These cellular grafts can be conveniently classified into cultured or non cultured epidermal cell suspension or cultured cells in sheet form.

- Noncultured epidermal cell suspension (NCES)
- Cultured "pure" melanocytes (CM)
- Cultured epithelial grafts (CE)

References

1. Falabella R. Surgical treatment of vitiligo: why, when and how. *J Eur Acad Dermatol Venereol*. 2003;17:518–520.
2. Prasad D, Gupta S. Standard guidelines of care for vitiligo surgery. *Indian J Dermatol Venereol Leprol*. 2008;74: S37–S45.

Excision with Primary Closure

4

About three decades ago, excision and primary closure was in practice to some extent to treat small vitiliginous area, but nowadays, it is hardly being practiced. In small segmental lesion, excision and split thickness grafting was also practiced. These procedures leave behind a definite scar. Even now, excisional surgery may be justified in small stable vitiliginous macules located in aesthetically insignificant areas. It should never be used on facial lesions except near hairline or within hairy scalp (Figs. 4.1–4.5).

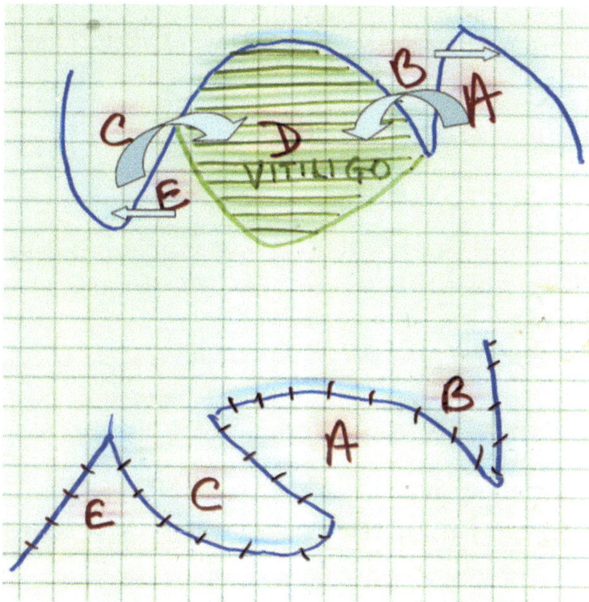

Fig. 4.2 Line diagram of rombus to w-plasty

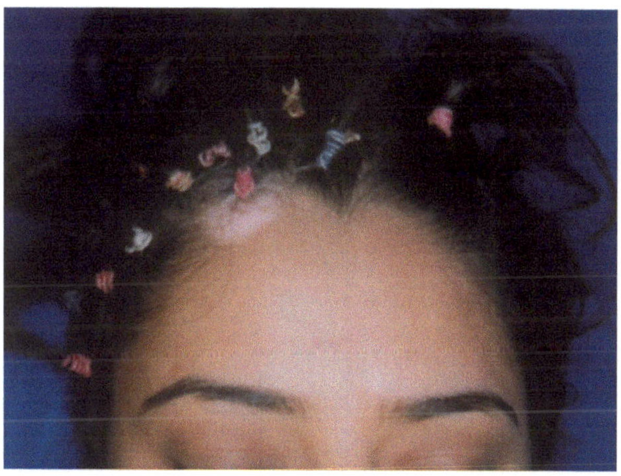

Fig. 4.1 Stable segmental vitiligo forehead

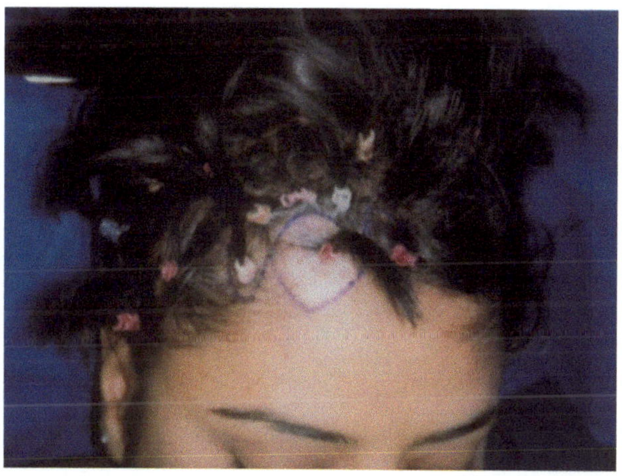

Fig. 4.3 Modified "rombus to w-plasty" designed for excision and closure of vitiliginous area near frontal hair line of forehead

D. K. Gupta, *Microskin Grafting for Vitiligo*,
DOI: 10.1007/978-1-84882-605-2_4, © Springer Science + Business Media B.V. 2009

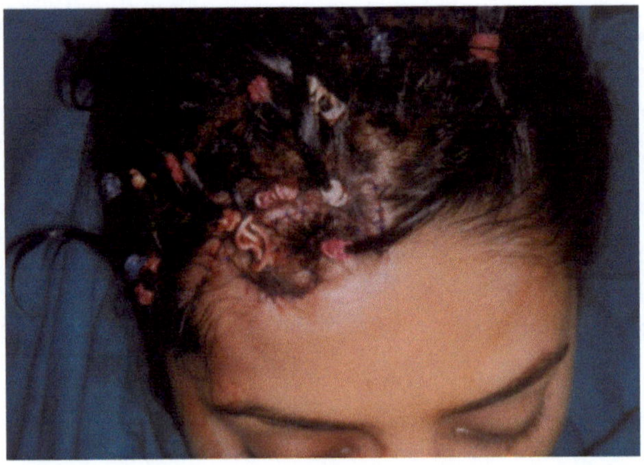

Fig. 4.4 White macule excised. Defect covered with transposed flaps

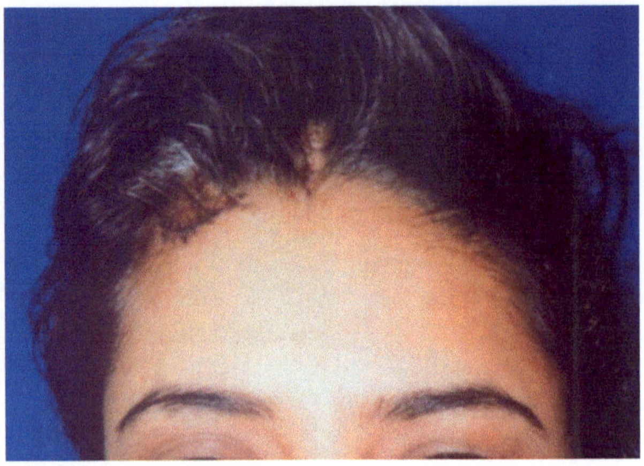

Fig. 4.5 Just after operation

5 Thin and Ultra Thin Split Thickness Skin Grafts (STSG-UT, STSG-T)

A split thickness skin graft (STSG) may vary in thickness from what is virtually a whole skin graft to one which is almost epidermal, and each has its place, depending on which property of the particular thickness is wanted.

Skin grafts are divided into two major categories: full-thickness skin grafts (FTSGs) and split-thickness skin grafts (STSGs). STSGs may be subdivided into thin (0.008–0.012 in. or 0.2–0.3 mm), medium (0.012–0.018 in. or 0.3–0.45 mm), and thick (0.018–0.030 in. or 0.45–0.75 mm) grafts.

Ultra-thin grafts (STSG-UT) of 3–6 thousandth of an inch (0.003–0.006 in. or 0.08–0.15 mm) are also used for resurfacing. There is less hypopigmentation of the donor sites after healing is complete, and reharvesting may be done if needed.

5.1 Split-Thickness Skin Grafts (STSG)

- Split-thickness skin grafts-blister epidermis (STSG-BE)
- Split-thickness skin graft-ultra-thin (STSG-UT)
- Split-thickness skin graft-thin (STSG-T)
- Split-thickness skin graft-medium (STSG-M)
- Split-thickness skin graft-thick (STSG-THK)

5.2 Thin Split-Thickness Skin Graft (STSG-T) and Ultra-Thin Split-Thickness Skin Graft (STSG-UT)

Since 1964, various surgical techniques and modifications have been used to treat recalcitrant but stable vitiligo with permanent and almost complete repigmentation. Behl[1] was the first to report the use of thin Thiersch's skin graft (STSG-T) to treat vitiligo (Figs. 5.1 and 5.2).

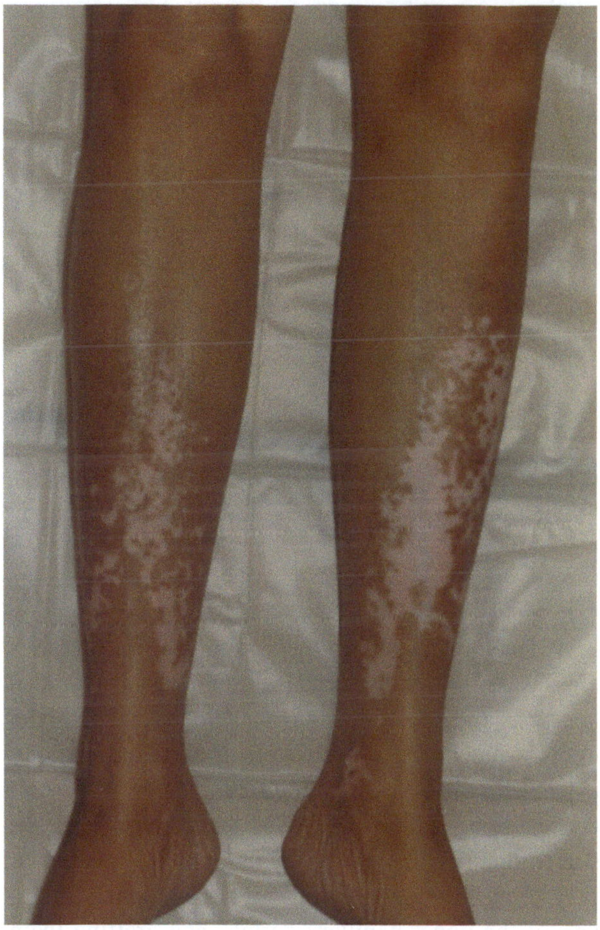

Fig. 5.1 Stable vitiligo vulgaris both legs

In 1993, Kahn et al successfully repigmented vitiligo lesions by a melanocytic transplant using ultra-thin epidermal sheets (STSG-UT).[2]

Several years ago, a successful surgical technique for treating depigmentation resulting from burn injuries

D. K. Gupta, *Microskin Grafting for Vitiligo*,
DOI: 10.1007/978-1-84882-605-2_5, © Springer Science + Business Media B.V. 2009

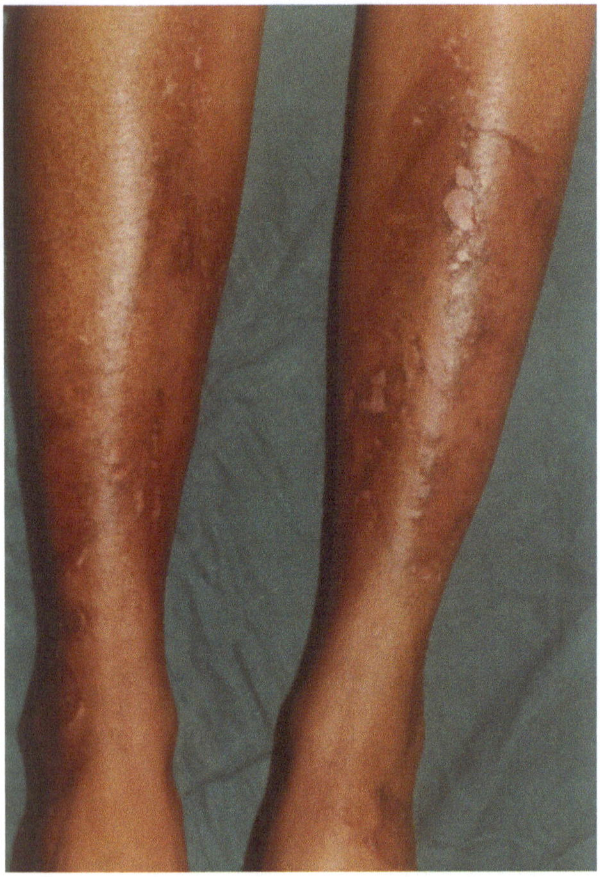

Fig. 5.2 Two months after thin (0.3 mm) split thickness skin graft (STSG-T) transplantation. Excellent color match but achromic fissuring is noticed on leg

was developed. The epithelium of the vitiliginous areas was removed by dermabrasion. The dermabraded area was then re-epithelialized with ultra-thin sheet grafts, which more recently were meshed and partially expanded. STSG involves the free transfer of the epidermis along with a portion of the dermis from one site to another. It consists of obtaining ultra thin or very thin, STSGs, consisting of the epidermis and a part of the upper papillary dermis, and grafting them on the denuded recipient site. The grafts are further secured with pressure and immobilization. Motorized dermatomes may be used to obtain ultra-thin split-thickness grafts, which may give cosmetically superior results compared to those with manual dermatomes (Figs. 5.3–5.6).

Good to excellent repigmentation was observed in 88% of the procedures. Scarring did not develop in the repigmented or donor site regions. The final color match has been good to excellent.[3]

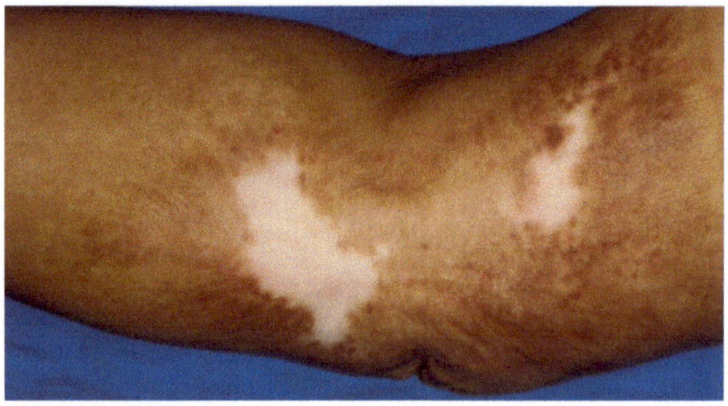

Fig. 5.3 Post burn leukoderma right – elbow

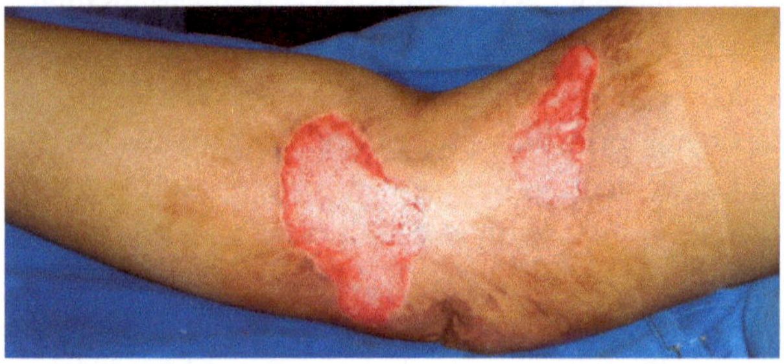

Fig. 5.4 Post dermabrasion raw area elbow

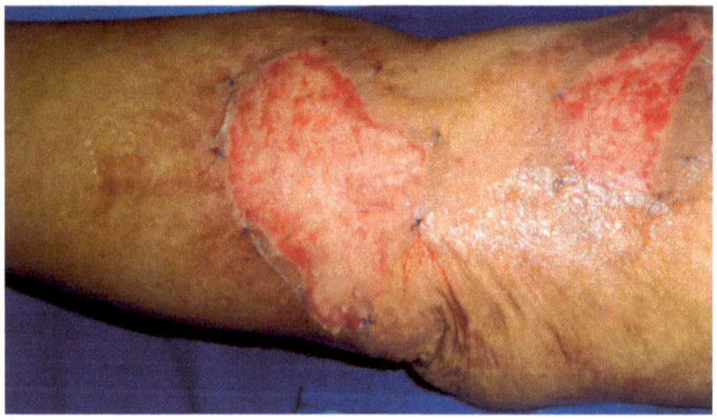

Fig. 5.5 Ultra thin (0.15 mm) split thickness skin graft (STSG-UT) applied over raw area and fixed with fine sutures to avoid graft movements

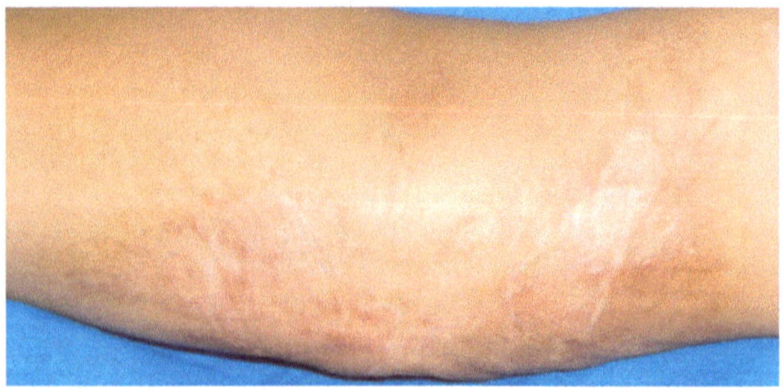

Fig. 5.6 Good color match after 6 weeks. Minimal perigraft halo is still visible

A split thickness graft covers the recipient area in a 1:1 ratio thus necessitating large grafts from the donor area. By using a Mesh graft expander[4] and increasing the size of the graft by 4 times, we were able to cover large areas with smaller grafts from donor areas. The advantage of the graft expander is that, there is no tissue damage and it adapts to a wrinkled or irregular surface. But this leaves behind ugly mesh graft pattern on the vitiliginous area which none of the patient would like to accept.

Machine-meshing a split skin graft,[5] gives it a three-dimensional flexibility that enables it to conform to irregular and concave surfaces without fixation. The drainage of fluid through the slit-like perforations prevents hematoma formation and permits the graft to be applied to an actively bleeding wound. Rapid firm adhesion occurs, allowing early mobilization. By ensuring that the skin is applied without expansion, excellent cosmetic results can be achieved. This method has the advantage of treating a relatively large area in a short period of time.

STSG has been used for the treatment of vitiligo for over three decades, but it did not gain popularity because of certain disadvantages. *Disadvantages*: include "stuck-on" or "tire patch" appearance, curling of the border with beaded appearance, color mismatch, milia, perigraft halo of depigmentation, and donor site scarring. Opting for ultra thin graft rather than thin graft, minimizes the above disadvantages.

The STSG-T is a simple, outpatient procedure performed under local anesthesia resulting in an excellent color match on a long-term follow-up. This technique can be used over any part of the body, including the hair-bearing areas, without compromising the end results.[6]

Repigmentation rates were 25–65% in the suction blister technique and 90% in the thin split-thickness graft technique ($p < 0.001$). The thin split-thickness graft technique is superior to the suction blister technique in treating vitiligo.[7]

Phototherapy using ultraviolet A (UVA) bulbs in combination with psoralen was used postoperatively, immediately after grafting of skin onto recipient sites.[8] In spite of reactivation of depigmentary effects at grafted areas, phototherapy acted as a stimulator for melanocytic proliferation and function and as an immunosuppressant, halting the melanocytic destructive process. The application of UVA phototherapy resulted in successful treatment in the patients receiving it.

Thin epidermal sheets, obtained by a high-speed air-driven dermatome, were used to repigment white areas in 19 patients with vitiligo and one boy with piebaldism. In the depigmented skin to be treated, the epidermis was removed by a rotating diamond fraise under topical and/or local anesthesia injections. The method was used on most parts of the body, including the eyelids and genitalia. The maximum total area treated on each occasion was 190 cm^2. Excellent results could be obtained if the vitiligo had been stable and had not increased or spread anywhere during the last 2 years. Lack of immobilization could explain a poor result in some areas. The donor area on the buttocks healed quickly without depigmentation. In the transplanted area milia were observed in the first 6 months. No scarring was seen. The technique has a niche in the treatment of depigmented skin, especially in larger areas.[9]

Vitiligo repigmentation induced by cutaneous grafts from the gluteal region and stimulation with UV and trisoralen. The extent of repigmentation achieved with this method was greater than the published data. We suppose that the stimulation with trisoralen over a cutaneous graft from a donor area not exposed to sunlight is more effective. This simple method is a good alternative for treatment of localized vitiligo.[10]

Modified Thiersh grafting,[11] in which psoralen without UVA or solar radiation was used successfully, is described.

A case is reported where overgrafting[12] was done for leukoderma of the lower lip. One and one-half year follow-up shows uniform color match of the overgrafted area.

References

1. Behl PN. Treatment of vitiligo with homologous thin Thiersch's skin grafts. *Curr Med Pract.* 1964;8:218–221.
2. Kahn AM, Cohen MJ, Kaplan L. Vitiligo: treatment by dermabrasion and epithelial sheet grafting - a preliminary report. *J Am Acad Dermatol.* 1993;28:773–774.
3. Kahn AM, Cohen MJ. Repigmentation in vitiligo patients. Melanocyte transfer via ultra-thin grafts. *Dermatol Surg.* 1998;24:365–367.
4. Srinivas CR, Rai R, Kumar PU. Meshed split skin graft for extensive vitiligo. *Indian J Dermatol Venereal Leprol.* 2004; 70:165–167.
5. Davison PM, Batchelor AG, Lewis-Smith PA. The properties and uses of non-expanded machine-meshed skin grafts. *Br J Plast Surg.* 1986;39(4):462–468.

6. Agrawal K, Agrawal A. Vitiligo: repigmentation with dermabrasion and thin split-thickness skin graft. *Dermatol Surg*. 1995;21:295–300.
7. Ozdemir M, Cetinkale O, Wolf R, Kotoğyan A, Mat C, Tüzün B, Tüzün Y. Comparison of two surgical approaches for treating vitiligo: a preliminary study. *Int J Dermatol*. 2002;41:135–138.
8. Sherif SA, Hamza AR, Hosam El-Din W, El-Domyati M. Epithelial grafting for vitiligo requires ultraviolet A phototherapy to increase success rate. *J Cosmet Dermatol*. 2007; 6(2):119–124.
9. Olsson MJ, Juhlin L. Epidermal sheet grafts for repigmentation of vitiligo and piebaldism, with a review of surgical techniques. *Acta Derm Venereol*. 1997;77(6):463–466.
10. Machado Filho CD, Bouro Neto JB. [Skin implants in vitiligo] *Med Cutan Ibero Lat Am*. 1985;13(3):243–246.
11. Bose SK. Modified Thiersch grafting in stable vitiligo. *J Dermatol*. 1996;23(5):362–364.
12. Chitale VR. Overgrafting for leukoderma of the lower lip: a new application of an already established method. *Ann Plast Surg*. 1991;26 (3):289–290.

Split Thickness Skin Graft-Suction Blister Epidermis (STSG-BE)

6

In 1971, Falabella, described the suction blister technique for repigmentation through melanocyte transplantation.[1]

I classify suction blister graft, a type of ultra thin split thickness skin graft that has pure epidermis. Basically, it is a technique by which epidermis is separated from the dermis, which cannot otherwise be removed by any of the cutting dermatome. Here dermal-epidermal separation can be achieved by the equipment which creates vacuum.

This procedure consists of obtaining very thin skin grafts consisting of only the epidermis (roofs of suction blisters). A physiological split is made at the dermoepidermal junction by the application of prolonged suction for 1.5–2 hours at a negative pressure of −200 to −500 mmHg to the donor site. Equipment needed, includes suction cups, suction apparatus and motorized dermabrader with diamond fraise/wire brush. The recipient site is dermabraded by using a motorized dermabrader and then blister epidermis grafts are applied to the dermabraded recipient site. The graft may fall off in a period of a week to ten days (Figs. 6.1–6.8).

Alternatively, the recipient site may be denuded by an Erbium: YAG or carbon dioxide (CO_2) Laser.

Up to now, results are promising. In this method, spreading of the epidermal graft to its maximum size and its accurate transferral onto the recipient area are important steps. However, the graft produced by this method is so thin and soft that it wrinkles and curls frequently, making spreading and transportation to the recipient site cumbersome. It had been found that the use of plain fine woven gauze[2] (muslin tulle gras) makes harvesting and transportation of donor grafts technically simple and effective.

According to a systematic review,[3,4] suction blister and split-thickness skin grafting have the highest rates of success (87%), while the average success rates for other methods varied from 13 to 53%. Punch grafting

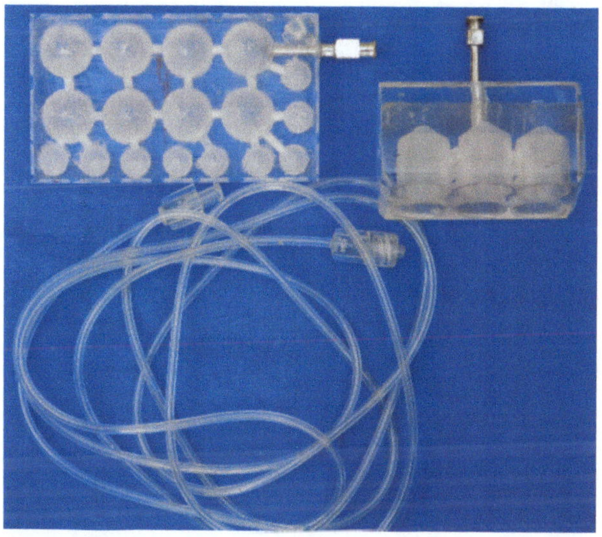

Fig. 6.1 Suction blister grafting: suction device with connected cups of various diameters (16 and 10 mm) and pressure connecting tube

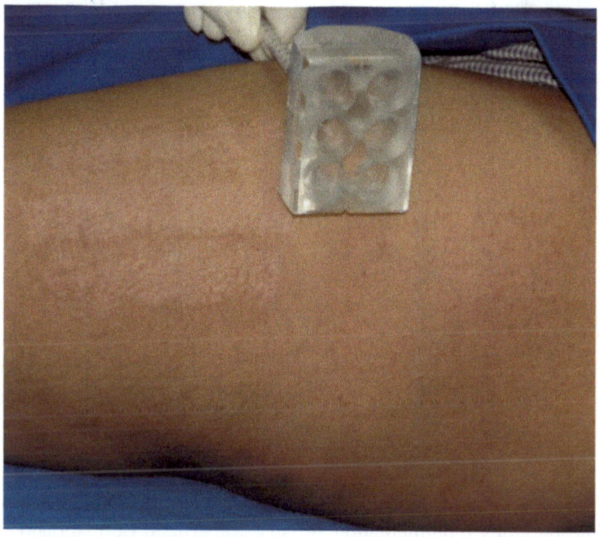

Fig. 6.2 Suction blister grafting: a suction device with six 16 mm inter connected cups

D. K. Gupta, *Microskin Grafting for Vitiligo*,
DOI: 10.1007/978-1-84882-605-2_6, © Springer Science + Business Media B.V. 2009

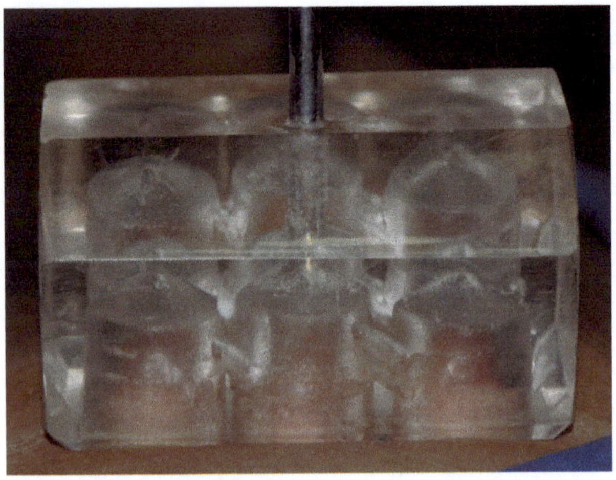

Fig. 6.3 Suction blister device applied on the lateral aspect of thigh by vacuum at –200 to –300 mmHg for 1–2 hours. Blister starts developing at about 1 hour and can be seen through the transparent cups

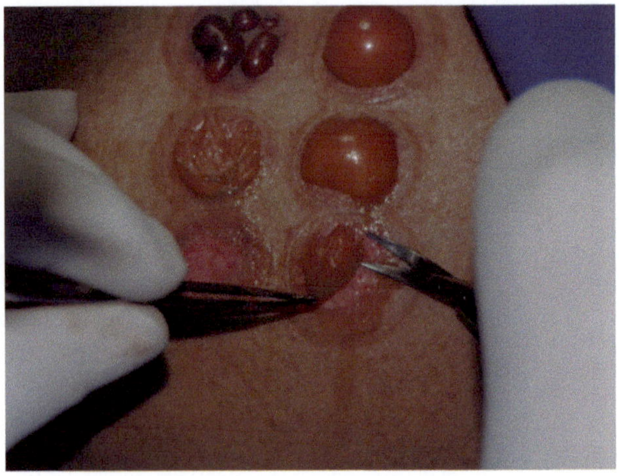

Fig. 6.5 Epidermal blister graft cut carefully with the help of iris scissor

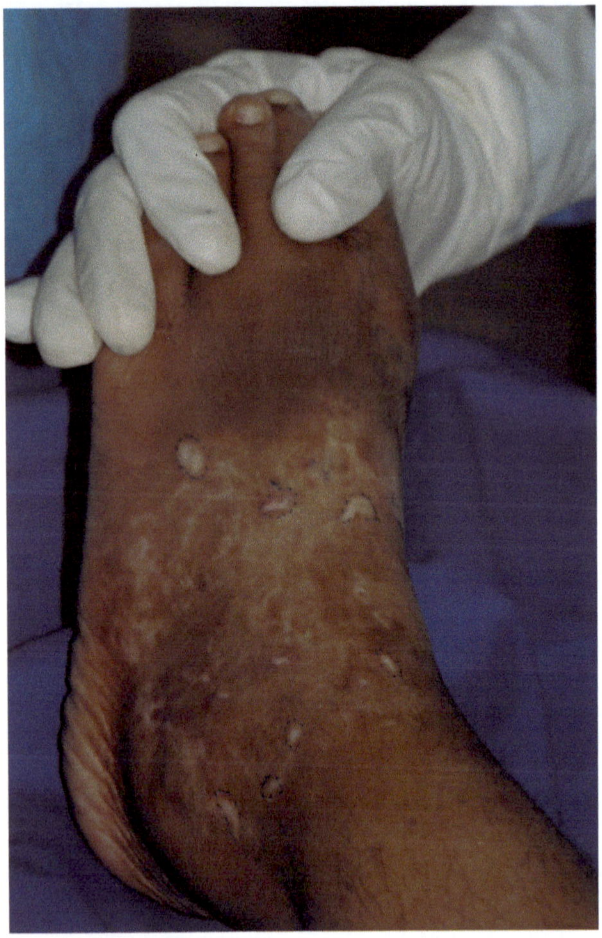

Fig. 6.4 Residual vitiliginous areas that were left behind from the previous repigmentation surgery. Superficial dermabrasion carefully done with the help of diamond fraise

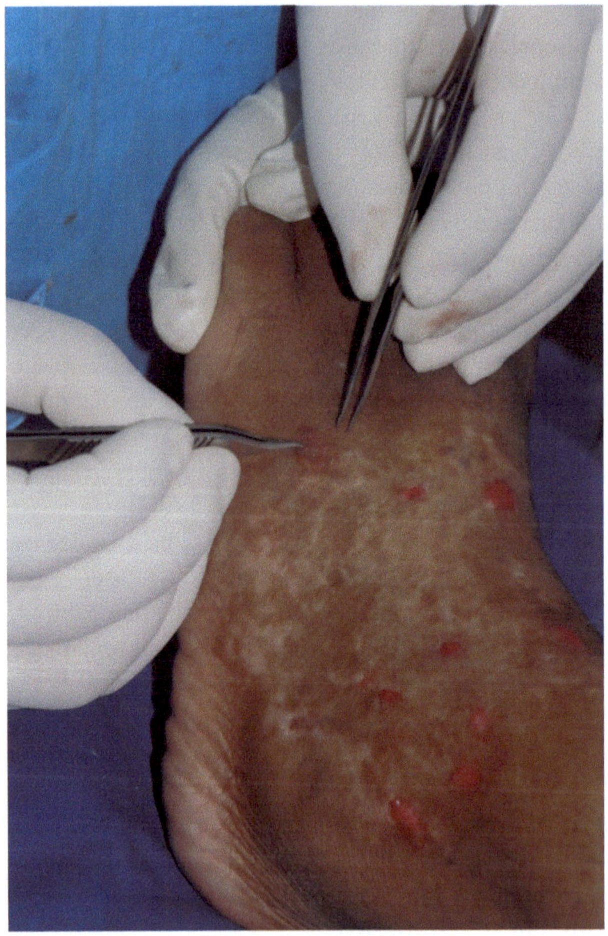

Fig. 6.6 Blister graft gently spread over the abraded area with correct orientation, keeping the raw surface toward the abraded recipient site

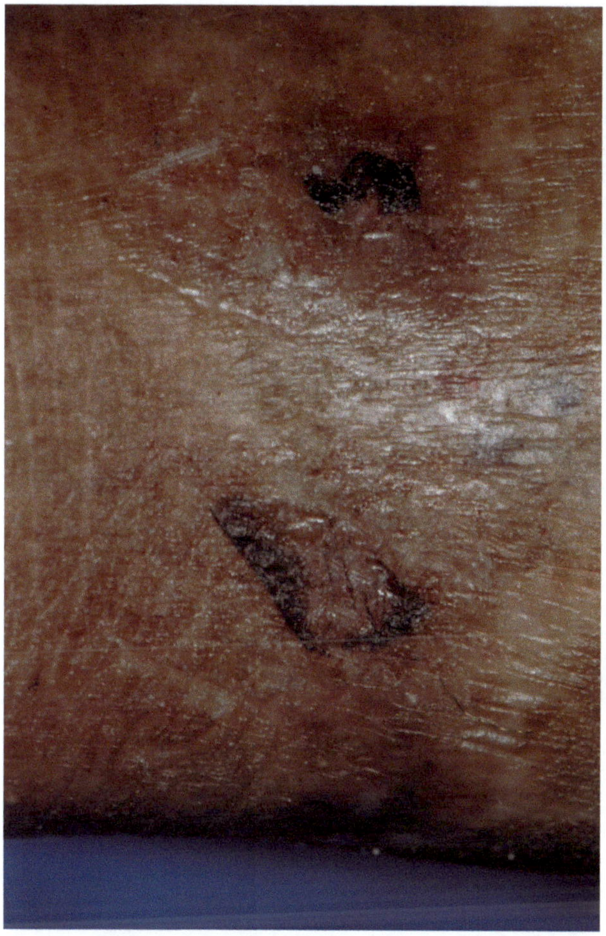

Fig. 6.7 At lower part of picture the blister graft nearly accepted. In upper part of picture the blister graft died and became *black* due to wrong orientation

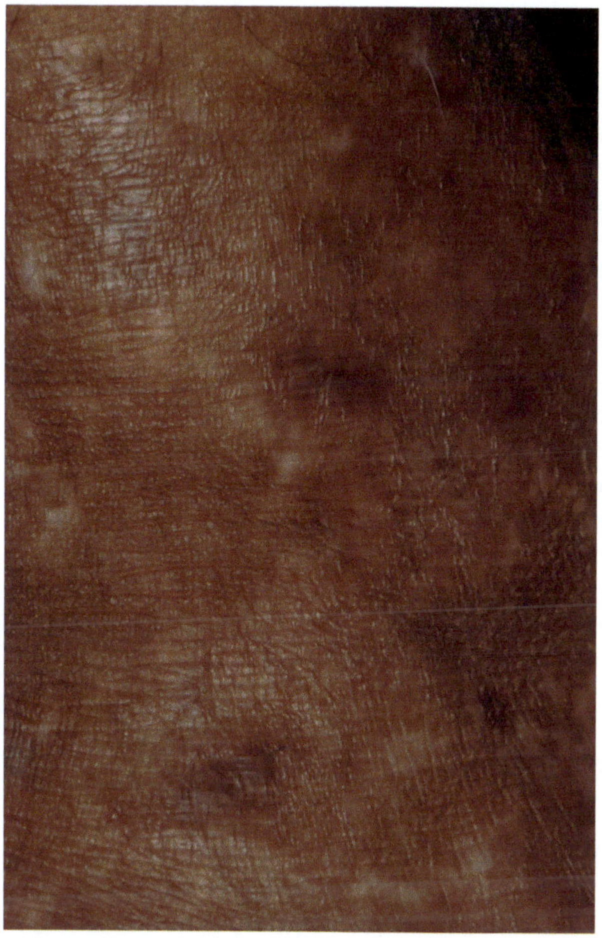

Fig. 6.8 Repigmentation is observed shortly after graft "take". Initially, the recipient area may get hyper pigmented as in the picture. Color matching with the surrounding skin takes few months

has the highest rate of adverse effects, including cobblestone appearance (27%) and scar formation (40%) in the donor site. Accordingly, it is also mandatory to appropriately select vitiligo patients in order to achieve a complete and permanent repigmentation.

In another study, repigmentation rates were 25–65% in the suction blister technique and 90% in the thin split-thickness graft technique ($p < 0.001$). The thin split-thickness graft technique is superior to the suction blister technique in treating vitiligo.[5]

The simple apparatus for raising blisters consisted of a cylindrical funnel or suction device with multiple interconnected cups, connected with a three-way tap, and suction was given by a 50-mL syringe or by a standard suction pump (200–300 mmHg.). The pressure inside the suction cup was retained by changing the position of lock of the three-way tap. The pressure was measured by connecting the three-way tap to a vacuum gauge. The apparatus remained adhered to the donor area because of negative pressure. The blister was formed in about 1.5 hours. The roof of the blister was grafted onto the dermabraded recipient site. The technique is inexpensive and easy and obviates the need of cumbersome and heavy equipment.[6]

Study[7] conducted for repigmentation of lip vitiligo by suction blister epidermal grafts shows complete repigmentation in 27 of the 31 lip areas (87%) in 23 of 25 patients (92%), in whom a follow-up for 6 months or more was available. Complications observed were persistent hyperpigmentation in 12 lips and reactivation of herpes in one patient. Minimal hyperpigmentation was seen in most of the remaining lips. The results of the meta-analysis revealed that the success rate varies from 32.5% to 100% with various surgical procedures. It is cosmetically more acceptable, as there is no abnormal keratinization, which is a problem associated with dermo-epidermal grafts.

No effective treatment has been reported so far for Naevus depigmentosus. A patient of naevus depigmentosus on whom the suction blister grafting was performed showed satisfactory resultant pigmentation.[8]

Two patients who had vitiligo with leukotrichia on the face and scalp were treated with epidermal grafting using suction blister after chemical epilation. Two weeks after the graft, they were treated with topical psoralen plus ultraviolet A (PUVA) therapy. Successful repigmentation of the skin with significant improvement of leukotrichia was observed in each of two patients.[9,10]

6.1 Micro Blister Grafting

Most of the time, suction blister grafts produce hyper pigmented patch work and color match takes a few months to a year. I have started micro blister grafts (MBGs) in place of blister graft to avoid drawbacks of blister grafts and at the same time increase donor to recipient area ratio. Correct orientation (epithelial side up) is a must for complete graft take (Figs.6.9–6.11).

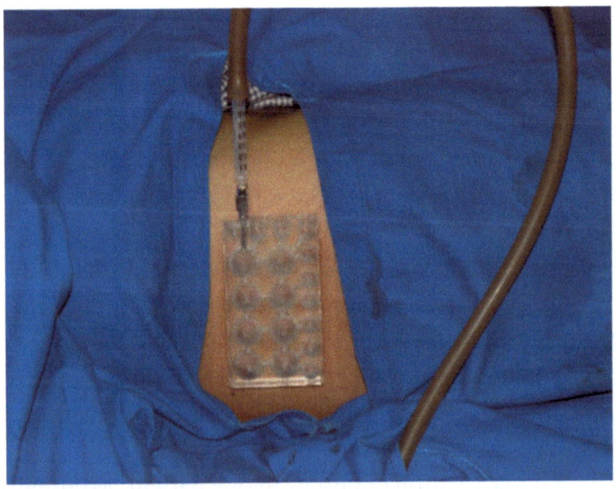

Fig. 6.9 Suction blister device held in place with vacuum

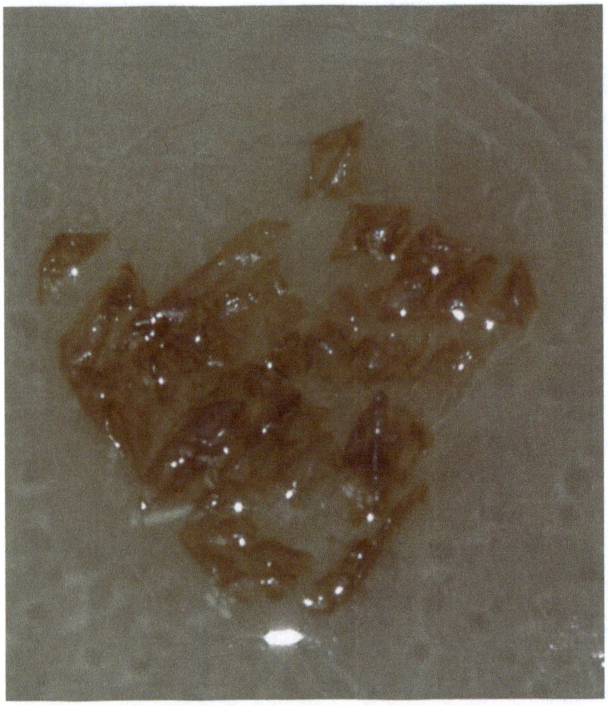

Fig. 6.10 Blisters are cut in the small pieces with the help of surgical blade. Micro blister grafts distributed evenly over the abraded vitiliginous area with correct orientation by reversing the grafts on vaseline impregnated tulle gras

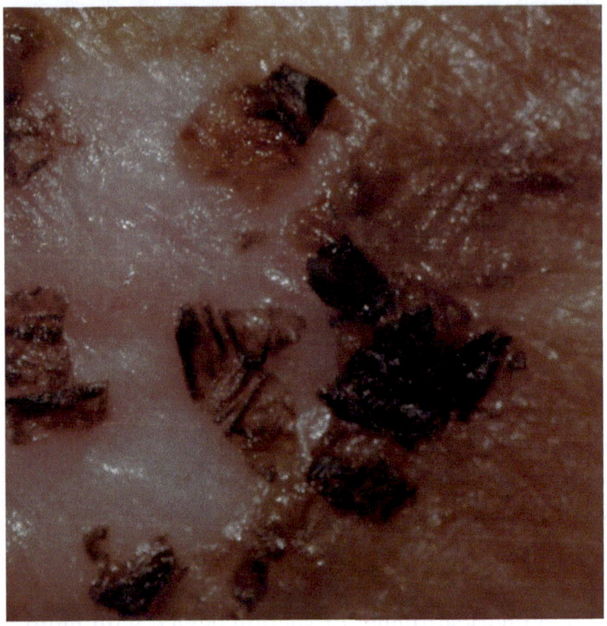

Fig. 6.11 Close up views of micro blister grafts (MBGs) "take". Micro blister grafts "take" on tenth day. Repigmentation observed from the margins of the grafts. Incorrectly oriented micro blister grafts and grafts outside the dermabraded area become dead and crusted out. Micro blister grafts with proper orientation start producing pigments

References

1. Falabella R. Epidermal grafting: an original technique and its application in achromic and granulating areas. *Arch Dermatol.* 1971;104:592–600.
2. Tang WY, De Han J, Lu NZ, Chan LY, Lo KK. Surgical pearl: fine gauze is a useful carrier for epidermal graft in the treatment of vitiligo by means of the suction blister method. *J Am Acad Dermatol.* 1999;40(2 Pt 1):247–249.
3. Njoo MD, Westerhof W, Bos JD, Bossuyt MM. A systematic review of autologous transplantation methods in vitiligo. *Arch Dermatol.* 1998;134:1543–1545.
4. Rusfianti M, Wirohadidjodjo YW. Dermatosurgical techniques for repigmentation of vitiligo. *Int J Dermatol.* 2006; 45(4):411–417.
5. Ozdemir M, Cetinkale O, Wolf R, et al. Comparison of two surgical approaches for treating vitiligo: a preliminary study. *Int J Dermatol.* 2002;41:135–138.
6. Gupta S, Shroff S, Gupta S. Modified technique of suction blistering for epidermal grafting in vitiligo. *Int J Dermatol.* 1999;38(4):306–309.
7. Gupta S, Goel A, Kanwar AJ, Kumar B. Autologous melanocyte transfer via epidermal grafts for lip vitiligo. *Int J Dermatol.* 2006;45(6):747–750.
8. Ravikumar BC, Sabitha L, Balachandran C. Naevus depiomentosus treated with suction blister grafting. *Indian J Dermatol Venereol Leprol.* 2000;66(2):89–90.
9. Kim CY, Yoon TJ, Kim TH. Epidermal grafting after chemical epilation in the treatment of vitiligo. *Dermatol Surg.* 2001;27(10):855–856.
10. Hann SK, Im S, Park YK, Hur W. Repigmentation of leukotrichia by epidermal grafting and systemic psoralen plus UV-A. *Arch Dermatol.* 1992;128:998–999.

7 Full Thickness Skin Graft (FTSG)

7.1 Punch Grafting

Falabella also introduced the autologous miniature punch graft technique in 1978.[1] In this procedure, punch grafts (of 1.0–1.2 mm diameter) are taken from donor areas over the thighs, buttocks, postauricular areas or the medial aspect of the upper arm. These are grafted into recipient sites in the sockets created by using punches 1.0 mm in diameter. To ensure a better fit, recipient punches are generally smaller by 0.2 mm than donor punches. Smaller sized grafts are used to yield better cosmetic results (Figs. 7.1–7.11).

Sockets are created in the recipient area (RA) at a distance of 5–10 mm and the harvested grafts are placed in these sockets. This allows the perigraft spread of pigment to cover the surrounding depigmented skin, the extent of which varies according to the skin color and site of the treated patch (more on exposed sites).

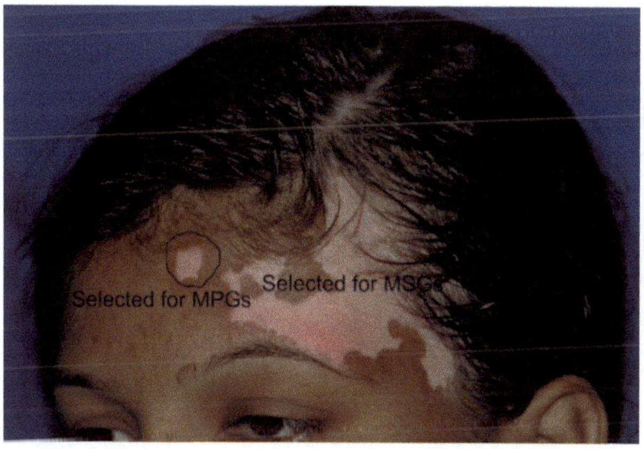

Fig. 7.1 A macule of stable segmental vitiligo on central part of forehead selected for mini punch grafting (MPGs) and rest of the area selected for microskin grafting (MSGs).This will also compare the surgical outcome at the same anatomical site by two different surgical techniques

After autologous miniature punch grafting, a remarkable repigmentation was obtained in 80% cases with 90–100% improvement. About 40–60% repigmentation was observed within 3–6 months in the majority (66.6%) of cases and near total repigmentation was

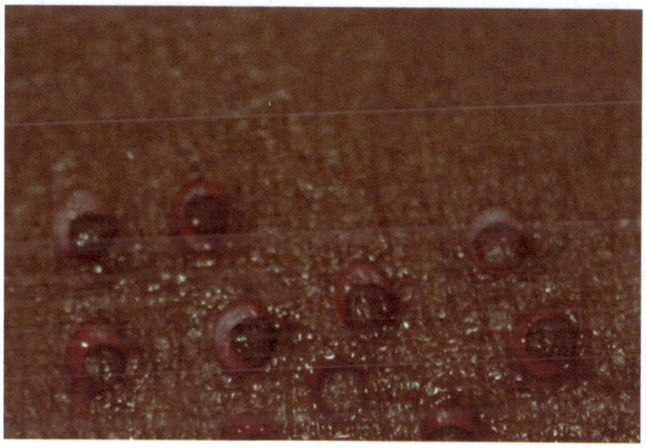

Fig. 7.2 Mini punch grafts (1.2 mm) removed from the gluteal fold

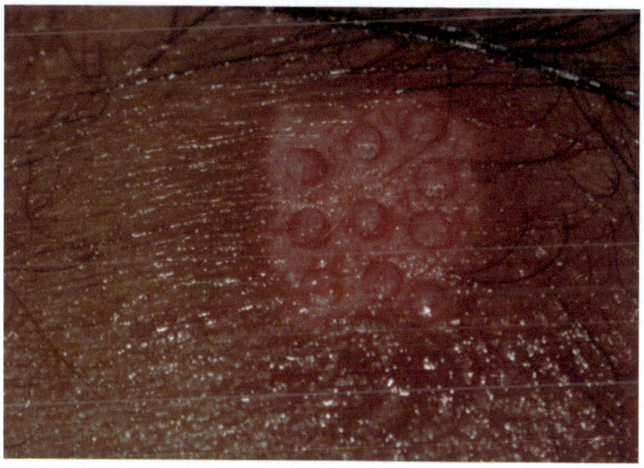

Fig. 7.3 One millimeter punch grafts cut from the recipient area (RA)

D. K. Gupta, *Microskin Grafting for Vitiligo*,
DOI: 10.1007/978-1-84882-605-2_7, © Springer Science + Business Media B.V. 2009

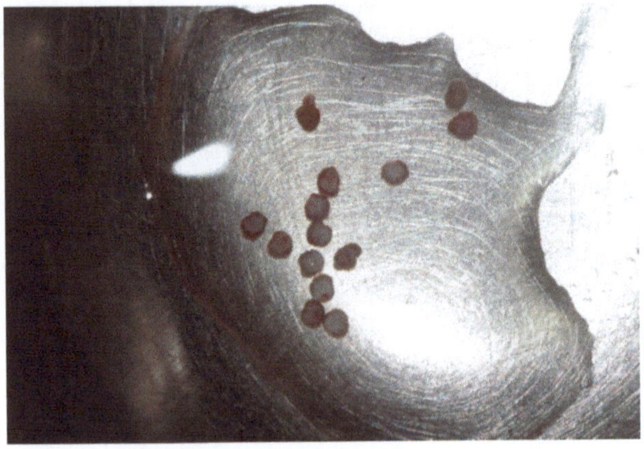

Fig. 7.4 Mini punch grafts (1.2 mm) kept in normal saline

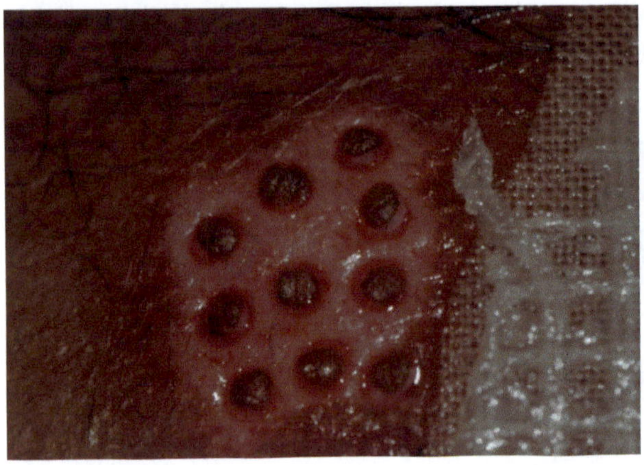

Fig. 7.5 Mini punch grafts placed in the punched out sockets of recipient area (RA)

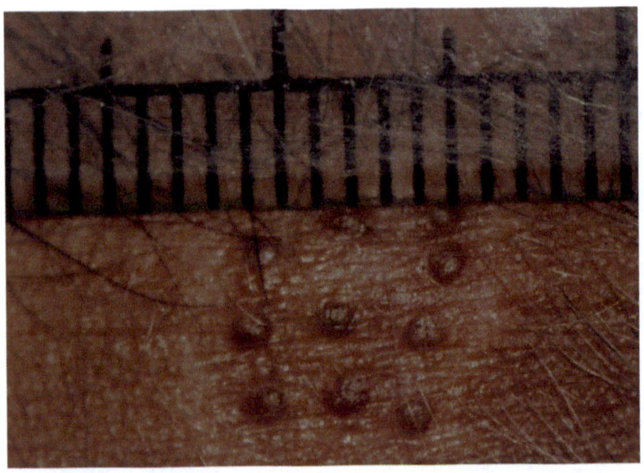

Fig. 7.6 Complete pigmentation achieved at 30th post operative day. Depicting the diameter of mini punch graft by millimeter graduated scale (1.2 mm)

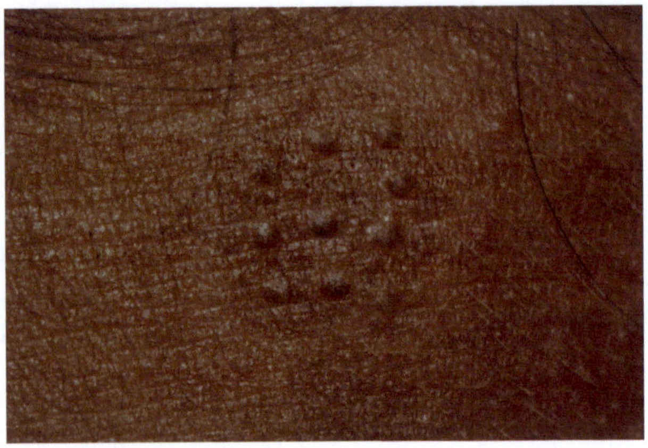

Fig. 7.7 Cobblestone effect is still clearly visible even with 1.2 mm MPGs (105th postoperative day)

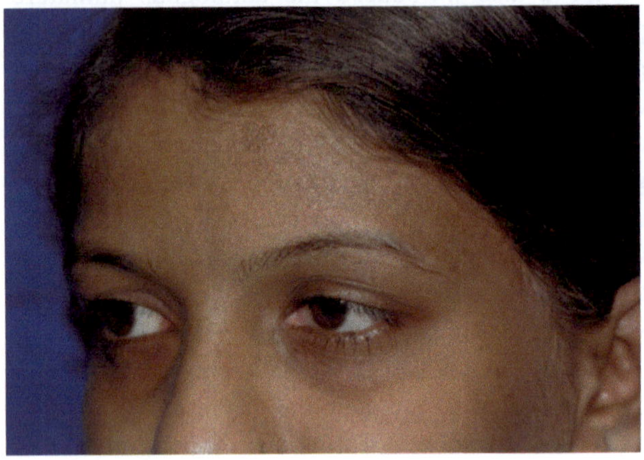

Fig. 7.8 One hundred and fifth postoperative day of 1.2 mm size mini punch grafting (MPGs) on central part of forehead and microskin grafting (MSGs) on left side of forehead and left temple region. Patient is bothered about the poor surgical outcome of MPGs on the central part of forehead

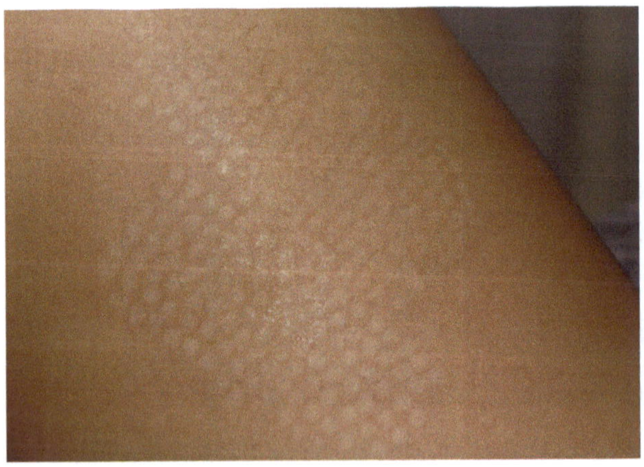

Fig. 7.9 Obvious donor site deformity noticeable on thigh with 3 mm punch grafts

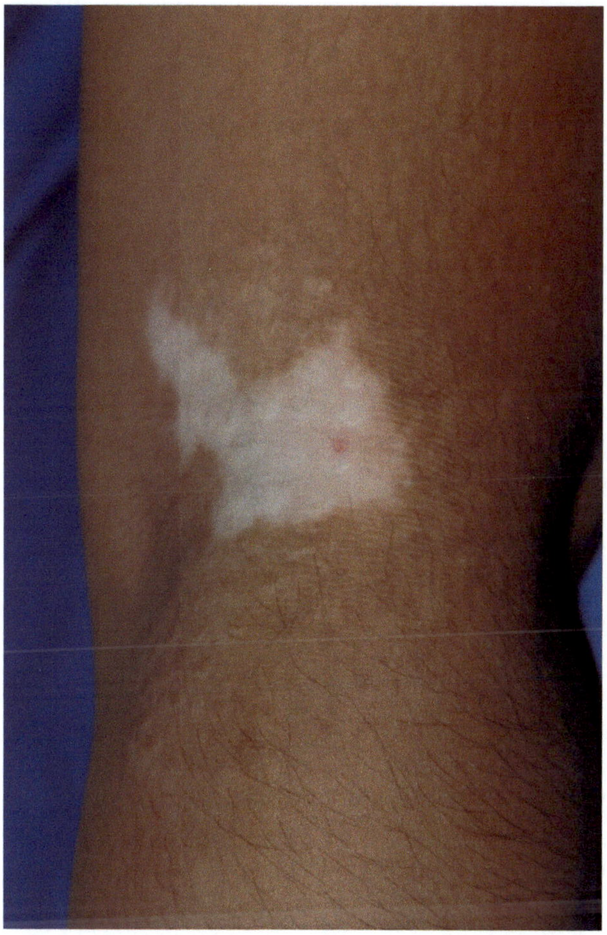

Fig. 7.10 Depigmented, but now stable, punch grafts planned for microskin grafting

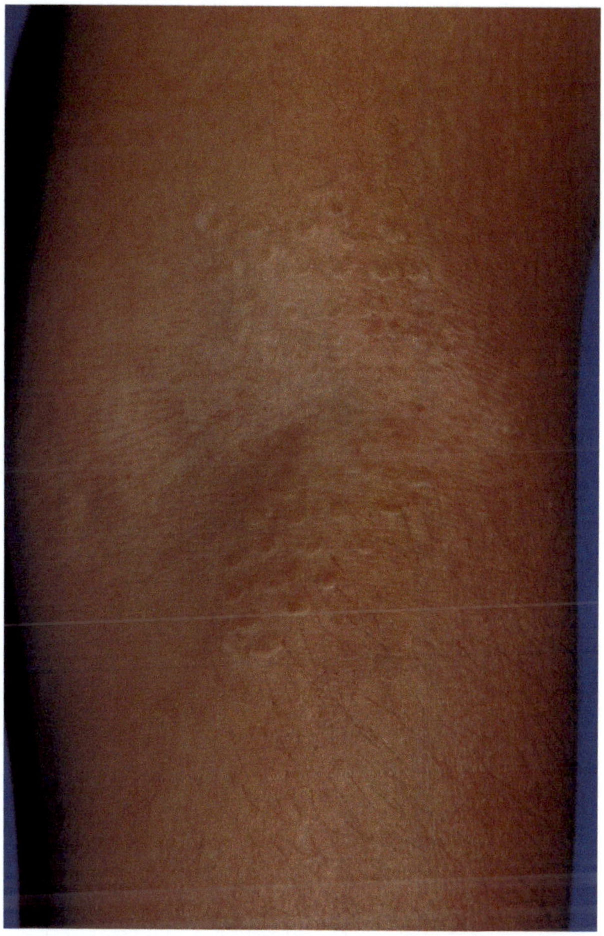

Fig. 7.11 Microskin grafting minimizes the cobblestoning of punch grafting and at the same time produces excellent color match

observed within 2 years. The maximum pigment spread (MPS) was observed over the face (cheeks) and neck, and the minimum repigmentation was observed over the left arm and right upper eyelid.[2]

Among various surgical therapies for the replenishment of melanocytes in recalcitrant and stable vitiligo, punch skin grafting (PSG) and suction blister epidermal grafting are the simplest ones. Literature is lacking for comparison of both. To compare the results of both surgical therapies, all patients were kept on psoralen ultraviolet-A (PUVA)/psoralen sunrays (PUVASOL) after healing of wounds. Results were evaluated after a follow-up of 4–7 months. The difference in both groups was not statistically significant. Cobblestone appearance (23%) over the RA and superficial scarring of the donor area (DA) (100%) were seen in PSG. No serious complications were seen in both groups. Both techniques are simple and effective, however, suction blister epidermal grafting gives cosmetically better and rapid results.[3]

A pilot study[4] was conducted to evaluate the efficacy and safety of pulsed erbium: YAG laser ablation of autologous minipunch grafted sites for the treatment of refractory or stable Vitiligo. Using an erbium: YAG laser to create graft recipient sites permits the survival of punch harvested grafts and the spread of pigmentation to the surrounding skin.

An evidence-based study[5] was carried out on the effect of narrow-band (311 nm) ultraviolet-B (NB-UV-B) radiation in 66 surgically treated patients with recalcitrant vitiligo, in whom autologous mini-punch grafting was deployed. Post surgically, they were exposed to a suberythemal dose of NB-UV-B (311 nm). The time taken for the appearance of repigmentation (AOR) in different regions varied between 14 and 32 days, with an overall average of approximately 20.6 days. MPS reached 12 mm with an average of 6.5 mm. The relationship between the donor graft area and area of surgical repigmentation was also calculated. Cobblestoning was the most common (31.8%) complication, but improved with time and/or interference. Punch grafting in combination with phototherapy (NB-UV-B, 311 nm) was found to be an easy, safe, inexpensive, and effective method of repigmenting static and stubborn vitiligo.

Patients with refractory stable leukoderma were treated with melanocyte transplantation. All patients received additional mini-grafts in areas of residual achromia. Surgical methods, followed by additional mini-grafting with 1.0–1.2-mm punch grafts, may be helpful to restore completely the depigmented defects when residual achromia, after treatment with the methods described above, is still present. The depigmented defects were 80–100% rectified in patients.[6]

Punch grafting followed by PUVA is an established therapy for stable vitiligo. The punch grafting followed by topical corticosteroid shows that the pigment spread with topical corticosteroid is comparable to that with PUVA. There was no difference in response to therapy in patients having segmental vitiligo, as compared with nonsegmental vitiligo. Cobblestoning, depigmentation of the grafts, infection, and graft displacement were the important side effects seen in some patients in both the groups.[7]

Of the various modalities of therapy available for the treatment of vitiligo, a combination of psoralen + ultraviolet A (PUVA) with autologous epidermal grafting appears to offer the best results. The erbium YAG laser can be used to prepare the recipient site in both punch grafting and suction blister grafting. All subjects with laser-assisted suction blister grafting showed a good response, compared with only 60% of those who underwent conventional suction blister grafting. The results obtained with laser-assisted grafting are more satisfactory than those achieved with conventional grafting techniques. We found that the repigmentation zones are larger (up to 9 mm in the former vs. 3 mm in the latter) and cobblestoning does not occur with laser-assisted grafting. Also, the procedure is precise, relatively atraumatic and can be performed rapidly even when covering vast areas.[8]

7.2 Minipunch Grafting

Minipunch grafting (MPG) and split thickness skin grafting (STSG) are common outpatient procedures for the surgical treatment of chronic stable vitiligo. However, there is a paucity of literature comparing the two procedures by the same group of investigators. To compare the two techniques in patients with chronic stable localized vitiligo, sixty-four patients with stable vitiligo of 6 months duration were randomized into two groups to be taken up for MPG or STSG in a representative patch followed by PUVASOL(Psoralen + UVA of solar origin) therapy for 3 months. They were evaluated 3 months postoperatively for the degree of repigmentation and side effects. In the MPG group, 644 grafts, 2.5 mm in size, were placed on a total vitiliginous area of 521.25 cm^2, whereas in the STSG group, 153 grafts covered a 1,489 cm^2 RA. Three months postoperatively, in the first group, 15 cases (44.1%) showed very good to excellent (>75%) repigmentation compared with 25 cases (83.3%) in group 2. Following MPG, 81 grafts (12.57%) were rejected. Cobblestoning was the main side effect, occurring in 13 cases (38.23%), and a variegated appearance was observed in 7 (20.58%) patients. The complications noted after STSG were achromic fissuring in four (13.3%) cases, graft contracture in four grafts (2.61%) in three patients, and rejection of seven grafts (4.57%) in one case; tire-pattern appearance in two patients (6.6%); milia formation in four (13.3%) patients; and depigmentation of the grafts in two (6.6%) cases. In both groups, superficial scarring was noted at the donor site in all cases, whereas hypertrophic scarring occurred in three (10%) patients after STSG. STSG carries a distinct advantage over MPG in producing excellent cosmetic matching over larger areas using fewer grafts, especially over the face and extremities.[9]

Vitiligo of the palm can be resistant to conventional treatments, and grafting is not routinely attempted because of some difficulties. The skin of the instep is an ideal donor site for palmer vitiligo.[10]

According to a systematic review,[11,12] suction blister and split-thickness skin grafting have the highest rates of success (87%), while the average success rates for other methods varied from 13 to 53%. Punch grafting has the highest rate of adverse effects, including cobblestoning appearance (27%) and scar formation (40%)

in the donor site. Accordingly, it is also mandatory to appropriately select vitiligo patients in order to achieve a complete and permanent repigmentation.

7.3 Hair Follicle-Grafting

Hair follicle-grafting[13,14] has been performed by a few authors for treating small patches in hair bearing areas and has been found useful in treating lesions with leukotrichia. A small strip of hair-bearing scalp is taken from the occipital area; single hairs are separated and transplanted into vitiligo patches 5–10 mm apart.

Dopa-negative, inactive melanocytes, present in the middle portion of the hair follicle and also in hair bulbs, have been reported as a source of pigment cells, when repopulation of epidermal melanocytes occurs. A melanocyte reservoir in these anatomical sites has been suggested. Scalp hair bulbs were transplanted within leukodermic areas in 10 patients with vitiligo. Repigmentation around the grafts was suitable for evaluation in four cases. Dopa-positive (+) cells were seen in the epidermal basal cell layer of the repigmented areas. Although these findings were observed only in a few patients, they suggest that melanocytes from the implanted lower third portion of the hair follicle (hair bulb) act as a reservoir in this anatomic location and are able to migrate and repigment achromic areas in vitiligo.[15]

Perifollicular repigmentation around the grafted hair was observed in 15 patients (71%) within 2–8 weeks. The diameter of the spreading pigmentation ranged from 2 to 10 mm during a 12-month follow-up period. In cases of generalized vitiligo, perifollicular pigmentation was seen in one of four patients (25%), whereas it was observed in 14 of 17 patients (82%) with localized/segmental vitiligo. Transformation of depigmented hairs into pigmented ones occurred in five patients. Single hair grafting appears to be an effective method for treating localized/segmental vitiligo, especially on hairy parts of the skin, including the eyelids and eyebrows, and for small areas of vitiligo.[13]

References

1. Falabella R. Pigmentation of leukoderma by minigrafts of normal pigmented autologous skin. *J Dermatol Surg Oncol.* 1978;4:916–919.
2. Sarkar R, Mehta SD, Kanwar AJ. Repigmentation after autologous miniature punch grafting in segmental vitiligo in North Indian patients. *J Dermatol.* 2001;28(10):540–546.
3. Gupta S, Jain VK, Saraswat PK. Suction blister epidermal grafting versus punch skin grafting in recalcitrant and stable vitiligo. *Dermatol Surg.* 1999;25(12):955–958.
4. Sachdev M, Shankar DS. Dermatologic surgery: pulsed erbium:YAG laser-assisted autologous epidermal punch grafting in vitiligo. *Int J Dermatol.* 2000;39(11):868–871.
5. Lahiri K, Malakar S, Sarma N, Banerjee U. Repigmentation of vitiligo with punch grafting and narrow-band UV-B (311 nm) – a prospective study. *Int J Dermatol.* 2006;45(6):649–655.
6. Falabella R, Barona M, Escobar C, Borrero I, Arrunategui A. Surgical combination therapy for vitiligo and piebaldism. *Dermatol Surg.* 1995;21(10):852–857.
7. Barman KD, Khaitan BK, Verma KK. A comparative study of punch grafting followed by topical corticosteroid versus punch grafting followed by PUVA therapy in stable vitiligo. *Dermatol Surg.* 2004;30 (1):49–53.
8. Pai GS, Vinod V, Joshi A. Efficacy of erbium YAG laser-assisted autologous epidermal grafting in vitiligo. *J Eur Acad Dermatol Venereol.* 2002;16:604–606.
9. Khandpur S, Sharma VK, Manchanda Y. Comparison of minipunch grafting versus split-skin grafting in chronic stable vitiligo. *Dermatol Surg.* 2005;31(4):436–441.
10. Kumar P. Autologous punch grafting for vitiligo of the palm. *Dermatol Surg.* 2005;31:368–370.
11. Njoo MD, Westerhof W, Bos JD, Bossuyt MM. A systematic review of autologous transplantation methods in vitiligo. *Arch Dermatol.* 1998;134:1543–1545.
12. Rusflanti M, Wirohadidjodjo YW. Dermatosurgical techniques for repigmentation of vitiligo. *Int J Dermatol.* 2006; 45(4):411–417.
13. Na GY, Seo SK, Choi SK. Single hair grafting for the treatment of vitiligo. *J Am Acad Dermatol.* 1998;38:580–584.
14. Sardi JR. Surgical treatment for vitiligo through hair follicle grafting: how to make it easy. *Dermatol Surg.* 2001;27(7): 685–686.
15. Arrunátegui A, Arroyo C, Garcia L, Covelli C, Escobar C, Carrascal E, Falabella R. Melanocyte reservoir in vitiligo. *Int J Dermatol.* 1994;33 (7):484–487.

Cellular Grafts

8

8.1 Noncultured Epidermal Cell Suspension (NCES)

Gaunthier and Surleve-Bazeille[1] used a noncultured autologous melanocyte rich epidermal cell /basal layer cell suspension in 1989. They injected cell suspension into blisters produced with liquid nitrogen. The scalp was chosen as the donor area. This technique was refined by Olsson and Juhlin[2] and further by Mulekar.[3]

According to a study conducted by Mulekar,[3] for the patients with a recipient area of >100 cm², a donor area of one-tenth of the recipient area was marked on the lateral aspect of the gluteal region. The area was then anesthetized with 1% Lignocaine. Skin was stretched and a very superficial sample of 200 μm in thickness (as estimated by a biopsy sample by a pathologist) was taken with Silver's Skin grafting knife. The thickness was adjusted by closing the screws at both ends. The superficial wound was then covered with sterile Vaseline gauze. The skin sample was immersed in trypsin solution, the epidermis separated from the dermis, and after some additional steps, a cellular suspension of keratinocytes and melanocytes was obtained, which was transplanted on the denuded recipient site.

The recipient area was abraded down to the dermoepidermal junction with a high-speed dermabrader fitted with a diamond fraise wheel. The ideal level was achieved when pinpoint bleeding spots appeared. The denuded area was covered with gauze pieces moistened with normal saline. Cell suspension was applied evenly on the denuded area and covered with collagen, which helps the transplanted cells to remain in place and provides an optimum environment for cellular growth and vascularization. This was then covered with sterile gauze pieces moistened with DMEM F12 medium. The treated area appeared bright pink immediately after removal of the dressing. The earliest pigmentation was noticed 3 weeks post surgery. Many patients showed hyperpigmentation, which gradually blended with the surrounding skin over 6–8 months. The donor area healed rapidly and soon became indistinguishable from the surrounding skin. Occasionally, the donor area healed with hyperpigmentation.

Repigmentation was graded as excellent with 95–100% pigmentation, good with 65–94%, fair with 25–64% and poor with 0–24% pigmentation of the area treated, as carried out by direct measurements.[3]

Patients with segmental and focal vitiligo can look forward to complete pigmentation of affected areas without scarring or cobblestone appearance. Repigmentation is likely to remain for a prolonged period, as observed by Olsson and Juhlin[2] in their study. The time required to complete a transplantation procedure is approximately 2–3 h depending upon the number of patches, anatomical location and the total area of involvement. In this treatment, the cell suspension prepared from donor area can be used to treat up to a 10-fold larger recipient area. Thus, patients with large vitiliginous areas can be treated in multiple transplantation sessions ranging from 100 to 300 cm² each, using a small donor area, which over a period of time merges well with normal skin. A biopsy of repigmented skin at the site of vitiligo treated with this technique showed an increased number of melanocytes as compared to normal skin.

After a strict preoperative selection for disease stability, transplantation resulted in repigmentation of at least 70% of the treated area in most actively treated vitiligo lesions. Repigmentation was primarily caused by the transplanted melanocytes[4].

To investigate a modified approach[5] in which noncultured autologous melanocytes and keratinocytes

D. K. Gupta, *Microskin Grafting for Vitiligo*,
DOI: 10.1007/978-1-84882-605-2_8, © Springer Science + Business Media B.V. 2009

are grafted on superficially laser dermabraded vitiligo lesions in a suspension enriched with hyaluronic acid, the cellular suspension was grafted on vitiliginous lesions previously dermabraded with a CO_2 laser. To improve the viscosity and fixation of the cellular suspension, hyaluronic acid was added. Three weeks after grafting, psoralen plus ultraviolet A (PUVA) or ultraviolet B (UVB) therapy was started. Residual leukodermic areas were subsequently retreated. Repigmentation was observed within 2–4 weeks and continued to increase for 3 months after treatment. In all patients, 85–100% repigmentation was achieved. A temporary slight color mismatch was visible in all patients. The most homogeneous repigmentation was obtained 5 months after treatment. This modified procedure seems to be a simple and promising treatment for larger vitiliginous areas.

In comparison with other surgical methods, the basal layer suspension method has the advantage that a fairly large area can be treated with the donor-to-recipient expansion ratio ranging from 5–10-folds. This technique requires a properly equipped laboratory and trained personnel.

This technique has now been simplified by the commercial availability of an autologous harvesting device (Recell). To cover wider areas, a similar system, called single cell suspension spray (cell spray), is available.[6] It contains expanded autologous cultured epidermal cells. Both these systems are expensive.

8.2 ReCell[7]

ReCell is a grafting device that allows skin cells to be prepared within 30 min. It also works by taking a skin biopsy although it is processed within the surgery. As the cells are not cultured and expanded, the procedure is limited to smaller wounds of up to 4% of the body. By this way, the skin tissue which is obtained from the patient is placed into the ReCell® apparatus. Then the skin cells begin to resolve through a special liquid in the apparatus and a cell suspension is provided. The treatment process starts with spraying this suspension onto the problem area by an injector. With a biopsy of 1 cm^2, an area of 80 cm^2 and through a biopsy of 2 × 2 cm, an area of 320 cm^2 can be covered by the healthy skin cells of the patient.

The suspension resulting from ReCell® contains a normal epidermal cell to melanocyte ratio and clinical studies have indicated the long-term restoration of color after the application of ReCell® cell suspension. These results have been supported with histochemical studies that confirm the presence of formed melanin and melanin precursors with the cells[8].

8.3 Transplantation of Cultured Autologous Melanocytes[9,10]

Melanocytes are cultured in vitro for 15–30 days by the addition of media and growth factors. Once sufficient numbers are present, melanocytes are detached from the culture plates and the suspension is transplanted onto the denuded recipient area in a density of 1,000–2,000 melanocytes/mm^2. The recipient area can be denuded by dermabrasion, CO_2, or an Erbium:YAG Laser.

Cultured autologous melanocytes were first introduced by Lerner et al in 1987.[11] Epidermal cells from pigmented areas of a patient with vitiligo were cultured in MCDB-153 medium, which supports the clonal growth of undifferentiated keratinocytes and melanocytes. The cells were grown on collagen-coated substrata. After the cells reached semiconfluence, the composite of substratum and cells was emplaced onto dermabraded vitiliginous areas as a graft. Re-epithelialization of the grafted areas was complete after 2 weeks. Repigmentation was evident after 1 month and continued over the observation period of several months. There was complete and normal differentiation of the graft, including a normal distribution of melanocytes in the basal layer. Ultrastructural studies showed a normal distribution of melanosomes in the melanocytes and showed keratinocytes that were indistinguishable from the uninvolved skin.[12]

Olsson et al, developed a technique through which we can multiply melanocytes, in culture, from a small specimen of normally pigmented buttock skin and reimplant them into depigmented sites of vitiligo. They reported four cases in which they have cryostored cultured melanocytes for 6–12 months, reimplanted them into vitiliginous sites of the donor after 1 week of reculture, and obtained optimal repigmentation. They now routinely freeze melanocytes left over after treatment.[13]

Autologous cultured melanocytes were transplanted to superficially dermabraded vitiligo areas in ten patients. Good cosmetic results were obtained in nine patients with stable vitiligo, but in one patient with new, increasing areas of vitiligo, no pigmentation was seen 3 months after transplantation.[14]

A pilot study conducted by J Phillips et al for grafting in patients with vitiligo, using cultured epithelial autografts containing melanocytes, gave disappointing clinical results, with pigmentation achieved in only one out of five patients. Irrespective of the fate of melanocytes grafted back onto the patients, they experienced problems in identifying melanocytes within these well-integrated keratinocyte sheets. This led them to explore the fate of these cells within these sheets in vitro, and to seek to improve their number and function within the sheets. They report that the introduction of a fibroblast feeder layer can improve melanocyte number within melanocyte/keratinocyte co-culture initially, but at very high keratinocyte density, there is a marked loss of melanocytes (as detected by staining for S100). Additionally, they found that keratinocytes not only downregulate melanocyte number, but also pigmentary function; thus, it was possible to identify melanocytes that were S100 positive but tyrosinase-related protein-1 (TRP-1) negative in confluent well-integrated keratinocyte sheets. In summary, their data suggest that keratinocytes at high density initially suppress melanocyte pigmentation (as evidenced by a lack of TRP-1 expression) and then cause a physical loss of melanocytes. The introduction of a fibroblast feeder layer can help maintain melanocyte number while keratinocytes are subconfluent, but fails to oppose the inhibitory influence of the keratinocytes on melanocyte TRP-1 expression.[15]

Advantages: The major advantage is that the procedure can treat unlimited areas; however, it is recommended that vitiligo involving >30% of the body surface area should not be treated surgically as chances of success are minimal in such cases.

Disadvantages: There have been some safety concerns about the use of cultured autografts in vitiligo. 12-tetradecanoylphorbol 13-acetate (TPA) used in the culture medium is a tumor promoter, making its long-term safety a concern. But recent availability of TPA-free and serum-free media provide a solution to this problem. However, this method is expensive and requires a tissue culture laboratory setup.

8.4 CellSpray XP

CellSpray XP provides a more rapid turn around time, 48 hours, and caters to more urgent emergency situations, although it can only be applied on, up to 30% of overall body burns.[7]

8.4.1 CellSpray

The CellSpray product is used where burns affect between 30 and 90% of the patient's body. Its application is limited to first degree burns, replacing the top layer of the skin, the epidermis. The technology involves taking a small skin graft from the patient, culturing (and so expanding) those skin cells in a laboratory for between 5 and7 days, then spraying the skin cells onto the wound. This differs from the alternative approach of skin sheets, which are grown in the laboratory and applied to a wound, 21 days after taking the initial skin cell sample.[7]

8.5 Cultured Epithelial Grafts (CE)[16–18]

Cells are seeded in a medium that allows co-cultivation of keratinocytes and melanocytes. A few weeks later, a cultured epidermal sheet is obtained, released by dispase and attached to petrolatum gauze. The recipient site is prepared as described in the cultured melanocyte transplantation section and the gauze is applied on the recipient site and dressed.

The major advantage is that cells are expanded in the cell culture to treat a large area. The technique requires special personnel and equipments and is expensive.

In nine patients with long standing, stable, and refractory vitiligo, autologous epidermis was cultured in vitro in H-MEM, but without growth enhancers or hormones and transplanted onto previously denuded achromic lesions. Repigmentation was achieved to almost 100% in three subjects, 60% improvement was seen in two patients, and 30–40% in three additional cases. Only one patient had almost no response. Long-term observations in these patients indicate that repigmentation obtained by this method is permanent. Transplantation of in vitro cultured epidermis bearing melanocytes is potentially effective to treat extensive areas of vitiligo, but this method is presently at an experimental stage.[19]

Under appropriate conditions, cultured epidermal grafts induce complete repigmentation of stable vitiligo lesions. The average percentage of repigmentation in 21 patients was 75.9% following Erbium: YAG laser de-epithelization and cultured epidermal grafts.[18]

Cultured epidermal autografting has been employed in a variety of clinical treatments including vitiligo management. Toriyama et al[18] successfully treated 2 patients with vitiligo using a short-pulsed CO_2 laser and by grafting the autologous cultured epidermis. Small pieces of uninvolved skin (2 × 1 cm) were taken for cultivation from a pudendal or axillary area and were expanded into two pieces of epidermal sheets 100 cm. Before grafting, the lesions were abraded superficially using a short-pulsed CO_2 laser with a computerized pattern generator. After successful grafting, repigmentation was visible within 1–2 months. One year after grafting, the skin color was almost the same as that of the surrounding normal skin. Thus, the combination of short-pulsed CO_2 laser resurfacing and cultured epidermal grafting is a powerful option for treating an asymmetric and wide vitiliginous lesion.

Plott et al[20] investigated a new technique in which normally pigmented epidermal cells from a vitiligo patient were cultured on a collagen-coated membrane in MCDB-153, a media that supports melanocytes and keratinocytes. The cell/collagen-coated membrane was used to cover a superficially dermabraded vitiliginous area. Clinical repigmentation, though incomplete, was evident in three of four patients in 4 weeks. Immunofluorescence and electron microscopy were performed on the grafted areas (involved and uninvolved controls). These studies demonstrated the reappearance of melanocytes and melanosomes within the grafted area. All three patients who were successfully repigmented retained their pigment at 1 year follow-up. Further investigation of this promising treatment for vitiligo is warranted.

References

1. Gauthier Y, Surleve-Brazeille JE. Autologous grafting with noncultured melanocytes: a simplified method for treatment of depigmented lesions. *J Am Acad Dermatol*. 1992;26:191–194.
2. Olsson MJ, Juhlin L. Melanocyte transplantation in vitiligo. *Lancet*. 1992;340:981–985.
3. Mulekar SV. Melanocyte-keratinocyte cell transplantation for stable vitiligo. *Int J Dermatol*. 2003;42:132–136.
4. Geel NV, Ongenae K, Mil MD, et al. Double-blind placebo-controlled study of autologous transplanted epidermal cell suspensions for repigmenting vitiligo. *Arch Dermatol*. 2004;140(10):1203–1208.
5. Geel NV, Ongenae K, Mil MD, Naeyaert JM. Modified technique of autologous noncultured epidermal cell transplantation for repigmenting vitiligo: a pilot study. *Dermatol Surg*. 2001;27(10):873–876.
6. Savant SS. Cultured and non-cultured epidermal cell transplantation. In: Savant SS, ed. *Textbook of Dermatosurgery and Cosmetology*. 2nd ed. Mumbai: ASCAD; 2005: 387–393.
7. Clinical cell culture's unique spray-on skin technology ready for world markets. *Bioshares*. July 25 2003;Number 32.
8. Navarro FA, Stoner ML, Park CS, Wood FM, Orgill DP. Melanocytes repopulation in full-thickness wounds using a cell spray apparatus. *J Burn Care Rehab*. 2001;22:41–46.
9. Czajkowski R, Placek W, Drewa T, Kowaliszyn B, Sir J, Weiss W. Autologous cultured melanocytes in vitiligo treatment. *Dermatol Surg*. 2007;33:1027–1036.
10. Chen YF, Yang PY, Hu DN, Kuo FS, Hung CS, Hung CM. Treatment of vitiligo by transplantation of cultured pure melanocyte suspension: analysis of 120 cases. *J Am Acad Dermatol*. 2004;51:68–74.
11. Lerner AB, Halaben R, Klaus SN, Moellmann GE. Transplantation of human melanocytes. *J Invest Dermatol*. 1987;89: 219–224.
12. Brysk MM, Newton RC, Rajaraman S, et al. Repigmentation of vitiliginous skin by cultured cells. *Pigment Cell Res*. 2:(3):202–207.
13. Olsson MJ, Moellmann G, Lerner AB, Juhlin L. Vitiligo: repigmentation with cultured melanocytes after cryostorage. *Acta Derm Venereol*. 1994;74:(3):226–228.
14. Olsson MJ, Juhlin L. Repigmentation of vitiligo by transplantation of cultured autologous melanocytes. *Acta Derm Venereol*. 1993;73:(1):49–51.
15. Phillips J, Gawkrodger D J, Caddy CM, et al. Keratinocytes suppress TRP-1 expression and reduce cell number of co-cultured melanocytes: implications for grafting of patients with vitiligo. *Pigment Cell Res*. 2001;14:(2):116–125.
16. Guerra L, Primavera G, Raskovic D, et al. Erbium:YAG laser and cultured epidermis in the surgical therapy of stable vitiligo. *Arch Dermatol*. 2003;139:1303–1310.
17. Pianigiani E, Risulo M, Andreassi A, Taddeucci P, Ierardi F, Andreassi L. Autologous epidermal cultures and narrow-band ultraviolet B in the surgical treatment of vitiligo. *Dermatol Surg*. 2005;31:155–159.
18. Toriyama K, Kamei Y, Kazeto T, et al. Combination of short-pulsed CO_2 laser resurfacing and cultured epidermal sheet autografting in the treatment of vitiligo: a preliminary report. *Ann Plast Surg*. 2004;53:178–180.
19. Falabella R, Escobar C, Borrero I. Treatment of refractory and stable vitiligo by transplantation of in vitro cultured epidermal autografts bearing melanocytes. *J Am Acad Dermatol*. 1992;26:230–236.
20. Plott RT, Brysk MM, Newton RC, Raimer SS, Rajaraman S. A surgical treatment for vitiligo: autologous cultured-epithelial grafts. *J Dermatol Surg Oncol*. 1989;15:(11): 1161–1166.

Part II

Microskin Grafting

What Is a Microskin Graft?

9

Ultra thin or thin split thickness skin grafts (STSG-UT, STSG-T) are minced into small skin pieces. The sizes of the small skin pieces varies from 0.2 to 0.8mm and the thickness varies from 0.15 to 0.3mm for the so called "microskin grafts" (MSGs).

Ultra-thin grafts of 3–6 thousandth of an inch (0.08–0.15 mm) are used for resurfacing. There is less hypopigmentation of the donor site after healing is complete, and reharvesting may be done if needed.

Fang et al,[1] evaluated dermatome settings from 0.002 to 0.012 in. (0.05–0.3 mm). First, with feeler gauges, he verified the dermatome settings. Second, he harvested the skin at various dermatome settings and measured the thickness histologically. He found that (1) the dermatome settings are reasonably accurate; (2) harvesting useful sheets at 0.002 and 0.004 in. (0.05–0.10 mm) is virtually impossible; (3) the variability of histologic graft thickness is enormous; and (4) a dermatome setting of 0.006 in. (0.15 mm) yields useful grafts. Further, graft thinner than 0.006 in. may contain no epidermal stem cells. If the graft contains no epidermal stem cells, it may initially take?? but then disappear over time, as the cells contained in the graft die and are not replaced. He no longer used the term epidermal autografting but rather ultrathin split-thickness grafting. To harvest these grafts, he merely set the dermatome to 0.006 in. (0.15 mm) and made all necessary midcourse corrections to obtain translucent grafts.

As early as 1895, Von Mangoldt showed that very small fragments of epidermis were viable, and indeed suspensions of individual keratinocytes have been used successfully for grafting.[2]

An alternative technique is to cut allogenic split thickness skin into very small fragments[3,4] and animal experiments have shown that particles of skin 200 × 200 μm may be used for grafting.[5] The limiting factor has been the development of a technique for generating very small fragments which retain their viability.

The study of Nanchahal[6] shows that fragments of split skin 40 × 40 μm can be used to graft granulating wounds. On an average, particles of this size would contain about ten basal epidermal cells. It is possible that even smaller fragments may be viable, but more sophisticated apparatus may be necessary to generate them by a relatively atraumatic technique.

No attempt was made to achieve correct orientation of the diced skin fragments, with the epidermal surface uppermost. Using skin particles about 1 mm in diameter, Nystrom[4] showed that improved orientation did not increase the healing rate. The explanation may be that the loss of more than half of the grafts (assuming random orientation on application) makes little difference because so many of the tiny particles of skin are viable. This would imply that greater expansion than that attempted in this study may be feasible. Alternatively, it is possible that the undulating surface of the recipient bed would result in at least, some of the dermal surface of the majority of the graft fragments being in direct contact with the wound site. This would be especially likely with very small fragments (40 × 40 μm). The maximum expansion achieved in this study was twenty-fold. This was not associated with an increase in the healing time. It is possible to mesh split skin widely, but this is often accompanied by a decreased rate of healing and partial loss of the graft, unless it is overlaid by an allograft.[7]

Apart from the greater expansion achieved by the technique described here compared to meshed split skin grafts, the final appearance was superior in that, the recipient site did not heal with a mesh pattern. The presence of a dermal component enhanced the long-term stability of the grafts.[8]

D. K. Gupta, *Microskin Grafting for Vitiligo*,
DOI: 10.1007/978-1-84882-605-2_9, © Springer Science + Business Media B.V. 2009

Cutting the thin split thickness graft into small pieces of skin is known by different names in the medical literature e.g. skin graft particles,[4] graft islets,[9] Chip skin,[10] seed graft,[11] MSGs,[12] etc. I adhered to the name "Microskin grafts" in the description of fine skin particles.

9.1 How Was I Inspired to Start Micro Skin Grafting?

For the first time, I used microskin graft in a case of post acid burn deformity on the face. These MSGs took well with rapid healing and good color match. This made me confident to use it in some other clinical problems like repigmentation of leukoderma/vitiligo.

It is invariably seen that a donor area of thick split thickness skin graft (STSG-THK) takes long time in healing by epithelization and ultimately remained hypopigmented and hypertrophied. In such cases, I used to spread MSGs routinely on the donor area. The donor area epithelized in less than 13 days and follow up of such donor area of patients showed good color match too (Figs. 9.1–9.3).

A study conducted by Zhang et al[12] showed that extensively burned patients can be treated with microskin grafting with encouraging results. The recipient area covered by MSGs ranged from 2.5% to 44% of the total body surface area (TBSA).The expansion ratio of the MSG, was 1:15 maximum. MSGs were distributed on the wound by floatation method. MSGs took well in patients when protected by split thickness homograft. I also got the idea from this study and became confident in using MSGs in repigmentation of extensive vitiligo.

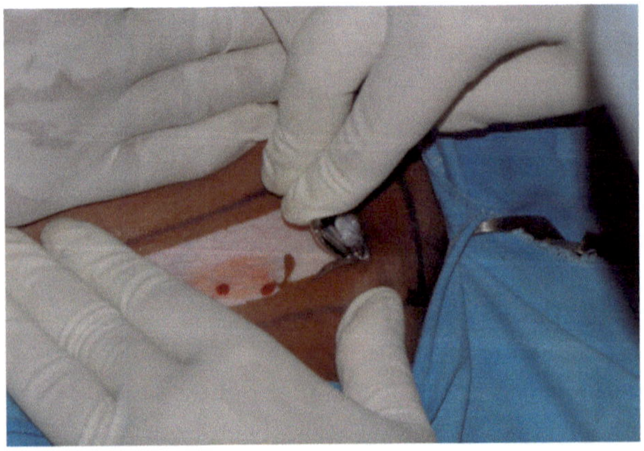

Fig. 9.1 Mixed full thickness skin graft (FTSG) and thick split thickness skin graft (STSG-THK) removal from lateral side of thigh with the help of modified razor dermatome

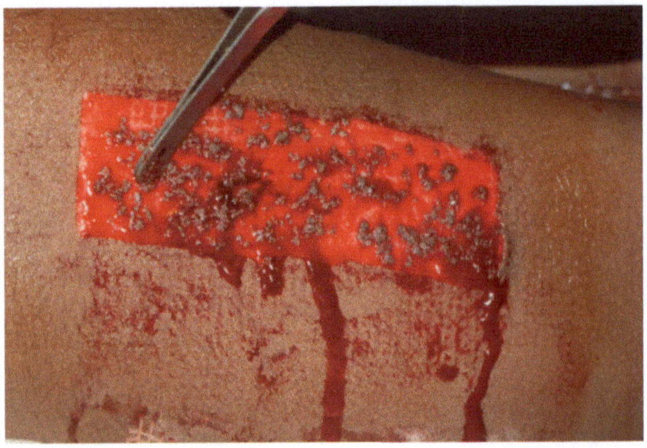

Fig. 9.2 Microskin grafts (MSGs) spread over the donor area following mixed full thickness(FTSG) and thick split thickness (STSG-THK) graft removal to avoid hypertrophic scar formation and depigmentation

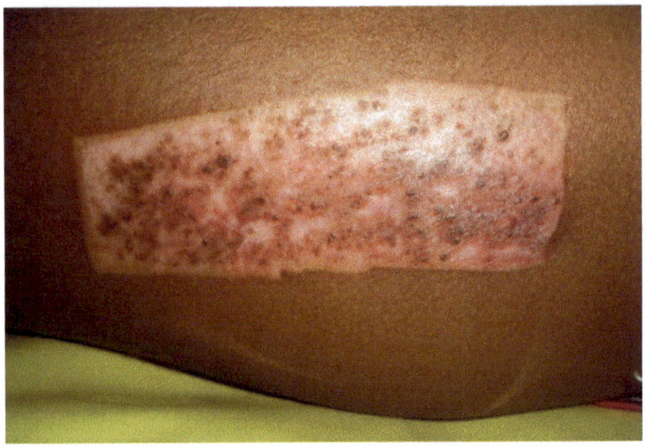

Fig. 9.3 Normal healing of wound within 13 days time and quite a good pigmentation of donor site on the 25th day

References

1. Fang P, Engrav LH, Gibran NS, et al. Dermatome setting for autografts to cover INTEGRA. *J Burn Care Rehabil.* 2002; 23(5):327–332.
2. Billingham RE, Reynolds J. Transplantation studies on sheets of pure epidermal epithelium and on epidermal cell suspensions. *Br J Plast Surg.* 1952;5:25.

3. Gabarro P. A new method for grafting. *Br Med J*. 1943; 1:723.
4. Nystrom G. Sowing of small skin graft particles as a method for epithelization especially of extensive wound. *Plastic Reconstr Surg*. 1959;23:226.
5. Blair SD, Nanchahal J, Backhouse CM, Harper R, McCollum CN. Microscopic split skin grafts: a new technique for 30-fold expansion. *Lancet*. 1987;2:483.
6. Nanchahal J. Stretching skin to the limit: a novel technique for split skin graft expansion. *Br J Plast Surg*. 1989;42:(1): 88–91.
7. Alexander JW, MacMillan BG, Law E, Kittur DS. Treatment of severe burns with widely meshed skin autograft and meshed skin allograft overlay. *J Trauma*. 1981;21:433.
8. Klasen HJ. *History of Free Skin Grafting. Knowledge or Empiricism?* Berlin: Springer;1981:84.
9. Rimdeika R, Bagdonas R. Major full thickness skin burn injuries in premature neonate twins. *Burns*. 31:(1):76–84.
10. Harashina T, Iso R. The treatment of leukoderma after burns by a combination of dermabrasion and "Chip" skin grafting. *Clin Transplant*. 21:(2):207–213.
11. Tsukamoto K, Osada A, Kitamura R, Ohkouchi M, Shimada S, Takayama O. Approaches to repigmentation of vitiligo skins: new treatment with ultrasonic abrasion, seed grafting and psoralen plus ultraviolet a therapy. *Pigment Cell Res*. 2002;15(5): 331–334.
12. Zhang ML, Chang ZD, Han X, Ziu M. Microskin grafting. I. Animal experiments. *Burns*. 1986;12(8):540–543.

10 Preparation of Recipient Vitiliginous/Leukodermic Areas

Treatment of stable vitiligo by repopulation of melanocytes with tissue and cellular grafts needs two basic procedures. One is the dermabrasion of recipient vitiliginous areas so that it can "take" the graft and second is harvesting of skin grafts.

10.1 Dermabrasion of Recipient Vitiliginous Areas

For the graft to "take" the vitiliginous area, it must be dermabraded by one of the following methods:

- Mechanical Superficial dermabrasion
- Laser dermabrasion(CO_2 or Erbium:YAG laser)
- Ablation by local PUVA
- Liquid nitrogen ablation
- Ultra sonic dermabrasion

1. *Mechanical dermabrasion:* Dermabrasion can be achieved using all the three types of abrading tool: the wire brush, serrated wheels and the diamond fraise. Diamond fraises are stainless steel wheels that have diamond chips of various coarseness bonded. Histological examination showed that the diamond fraise left a smooth abraded surface and the wire brush left an uneven surface. EMLA (eutectic mixture of local anesthetics) cream, usually used for skin surface analgesia, was tested as an adjunct to anesthesia in dermabrasion. EMLA's analgesic performance alone was insufficient in the sensitive perioral region, but it elevated the pain threshold and decreased the required amount of local anesthetic solution. In the past, dermabrasion was done using a small, sterilized, electric sander. In the past decade, it has become more common to use a CO_2 or Erbium:YAG laser. Laser dermabrasion is much easier to control, much easier to gauge, and is practically bloodless compared to classic dermabrasion. In the author's opinion, with little experience, the wire brush and diamond fraise do dermabrasion very fast with practically no friction thermal injury to the underlying dermis.
2. *CO_2 Laser dermabrasion:* Dermabrasion of depigmented area can be performed by using Ultrapulse carbon dioxide (CO_2) laser with a computerized pattern generator. The depigmented areas can be dermabraded in a short time; depth of tissue ablation can be well controlled; and a bloodless and smooth raw surface can be created by using a flash-scanned carbon dioxide laser. These raw surfaces sustain thin skin grafts well. The Ultrapulse CO_2 laser is particularly well suited for de-epithelialization in vitiligo surgery.

Laser-induced thermal damage on the graft bed measuring greater than $160 \pm 60\,\mu m$ in depth, significantly decreased skin graft take. Other deleterious effects included, delayed graft revascularization, increased inflammatory cell infiltrate at the graft-wound bed interface, and accelerated formation of hypertrophied fibrous tissue within the graft bed and underlying muscle. Ablative lasers developed for cutaneous surgery should create less than $160 \pm 60\,\mu m$ of residual thermal damage to permit optimal skin graft take and healing[1] (Figs. 10.1 and 10.2).

Dermabrasion followed by skin grafting has been used for treatment of depigmentation. The short pulsed carbon dioxide (CO_2) laser allows removal of the epidermis but leaves necrosis on the surface of the dermis. Two vitiliginous areas of skin were de-epithelialized, one by conventional dermabrasion and the other with a pulsed

D. K. Gupta, *Microskin Grafting for Vitiligo*,
DOI: 10.1007/978-1-84882-605-2_10,

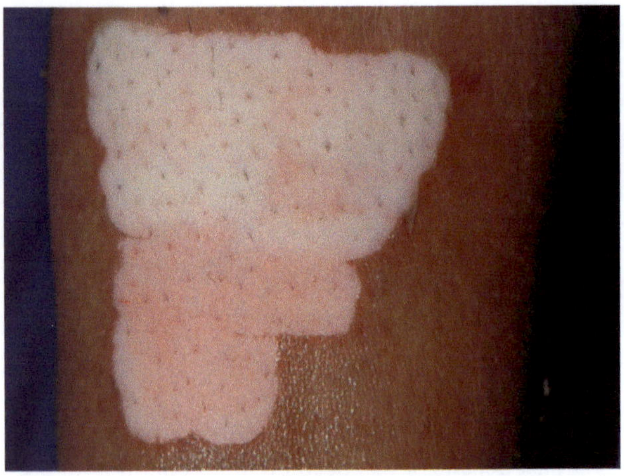

Fig. 10.1 Deep thermal damage in left upper quadrant by CO_2 laser ablation

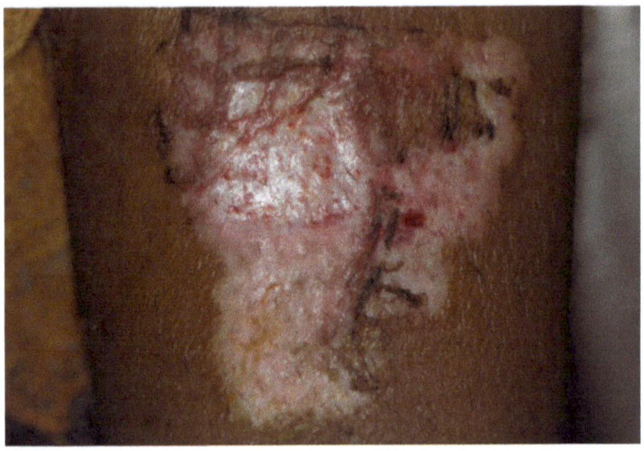

Fig. 10.2 Partial or no graft take in deep thermal damaged area by CO_2 laser ablation

CO_2 laser. Each area was biopsied for histologic study and grafted with a split-thickness skin graft. Histologic studies of the wounds were compared. The residual tissue destruction on the dermis of each area was quite similar. The skin graft take was excellent in both areas. The short pulsed CO_2 laser does not cause sufficient thermal necrosis on the surface of the papillary dermis to interfere with a satisfactory skin graft take.[2]

3. *Erbium:YAG Laser dermabrasion:* The erbium:-YAG laser can be used to prepare the recipient site. The erbium:YAG laser is an ideal tool for creating graft recipient sites, given its precision in terms of width and depth of ablation.[3]
4. *Inducing a phototoxic blister in the recipient site:* Topical psoralen, 8 MOP solution, followed by UVA in a higher dose prior to treatment leads to separation of the epidermis from the dermis. The epidermis can then be rapidly removed by using saline-soaked gauze. On the vitiliginous areas 0.075% of 8-methoxypsoralen was applied and after 10min the affected part was exposed to 10J/cm^2 of UVA in PUVA full body unit for two consecutive days before surgery. On the day of the surgery, the vitiliginous skin was erythematous with blisters over a few areas. The erythematous and blistered vitiliginous skin was rubbed vigorously with a saline-soaked gauze piece held between the thumb and index fingers to remove the epidermis. Areas of epidermis not removed by this procedure were dermabraded using a wire planing brush.[4]
5. *Liquid nitrogen ablation:* Production of blisters on the depigmented lesions can be produced by freezing with liquid nitrogen. Even liquid nitrogen, if used excessively, can cause severe inflammation in the recipient site, which results in hypertrophic scarring and post inflammatory hyperpigmentation.[5]
6. *Ultrasonic dermabrasion:* The ultrasonic surgical aspirator abrades only the epidermis of the recipient sites. This easily and safely removes only the epidermis, even on spotty lesions or intricate regions which are difficult to remove using a conventional motor-driven grinder or liquid nitrogen.[6]

Note: Mechanical superficial dermabrasion, CO_2 laser and Erbium:YAG laser dermabrasion are the best methods for dermabrasion of large vitiliginous area and are the methods of choice.

10.2 Eye Protection Be Worn During Dermatological Surgery

There is a substantial risk of a splash of blood coming into contact with the face during dermatological surgery for both the operator and assistant, regardless of the procedure. The risk of receiving a blood splash to the face may be substantially underestimated by dermatologists. The use of protective eyewear is advisable at all times, but particularly when using bipolar electrocautery, or when operating on high-risk individuals[7,8] (Fig. 10.3).

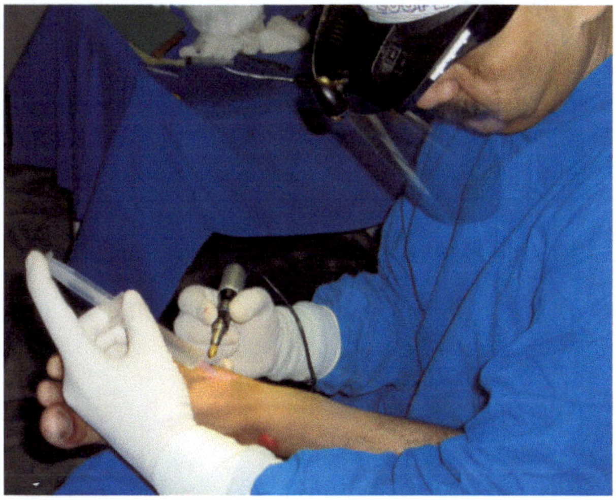

Fig. 10.3 Surgeon must use protective eyewear

References

1. Green HA, Burd EE, Nishioka NS, Compton CC. Skin graft take and healing following 193-nm excimer, continuous-wave carbon dioxide (CO_2), pulsed CO_2, or pulsed holmium: YAG laser ablation of the graft bed. *Arch Dermatol.* 1993; 129(8):979–988.
2. Kahn AM, Ostad A, Moy RL. Grafting following short-pulse carbon dioxide laser de-epithelialization. *Dermatol Surg.* 1996;22(11):965–967.
3. Guerra L, Primavera G, et al. Erbium:YAG laser and cultured epidermis in the surgical therapy of stable vitiligo. *Arch Dermatol.* 2003;139:(10):1303–1310.
4. Srinivas CR, Rai R, Kumar PU. Meshed split skin graft for extensive vitiligo. *Indian J Dermatol Venereol Leprol.* 2004; 70:165–167.
5. Gauthier Y, Surleve-Brazeille JE. Autologous grafting with noncultured melanocytes; a simplified method for treatment of depigmented lesions. *J Am Acad Dermatol.* 1992;26: 191–194.
6. Tsukamoto K, Osada A, Kitamura R, Ohkouchi M, Shimada S, Takayama O. Approaches to repigmentation of vitiligo skin: new treatment with ultrasonic abrasion, seed-grafting and psoralen plus ultraviolet A therapy. *Pigment Cell Res.* 2002;15:(5):331–334.
7. Collins D, Rice J, Nicholson P, Barry K. Quantification of facial contamination with blood during orthopaedic procedures. *J Hosp Infect.* 2000;45:73–75.
8. Kouri DL, Ernest JM. Incidence of perceived and actual face shield contamination during vaginal and caesarean delivery. *Am J Obstet Gynecol.* 1993;169:312–316.

Superficial Dermabrasion of Vitiliginous Skin

11

11.1 What is Dermabrasion?

Dermabrasion is a technique of skin resurfacing in which a high-speed rotary instrument with various abrasive end pieces is used to remove chosen layers of skin. The epidermis then regenerates from epidermal appendages in the deep dermis. The procedure can be performed with either a diamond fraise, which removes tissue by friction injury, or a wire brush, which removes tissue through microlacerations. The recipient area is abraded until tiny point bleeding spots are seen, which imply that the dermoepidermal junction has been reached. The denuded area is covered with a saline moistened gauze piece.

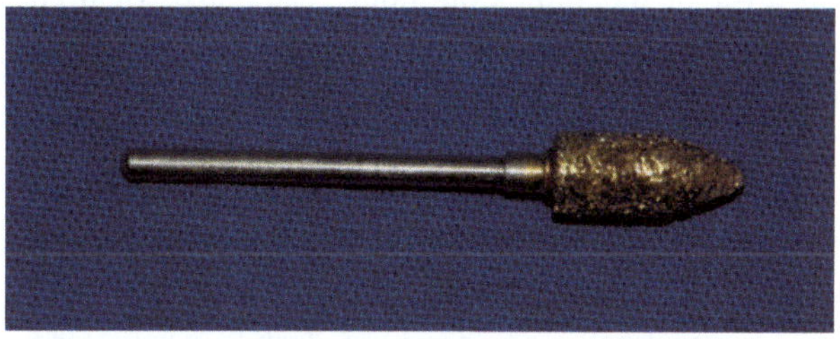

Fig. 11.1 Commonly used diamond fraise 17 × 8

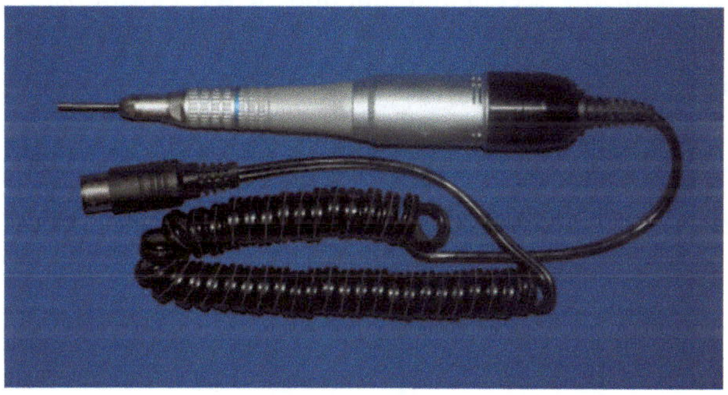

Fig. 11.2 Light duty electric hand engine used for small lesions. Dental Micro motor can be used

11.2 Anesthesia for Dermabrasion

The area to be dermabraded is cleaned with soap and water, 70% ethanol and painted with povidone iodine and at last, washed thoroughly with normal saline. It is anesthetized with use of eutectic mixture of local anesthetics (EMLA), infiltration anesthesia, nerve blocks and regional anesthesia. In extensive vitiligo, general anesthesia may be needed.

11.3 Mechanical Dermabrasion Tools

11.3.1 Dermabrader

The dermabrader consists of an electric hand engine with a high-speed rotary motor and an interchangeable abrading end piece (Figs. 11.1 and 11.2). The surgeon controls the speed with a foot pedal. Pressure exerted on the hand piece and the revolutions per minute of the hand piece are the two most important variables. Avoiding excessive pressure on the hand piece is important because this can result in gouging. Suggested rotational speeds of 12,000–15,000 rpm for the abrading heads result in controlled gradual planing of the treated surface.

11.4 Diamond Fraises

Diamond fraises come in different shapes and sizes like cone, dome, pear, bullet and mini bullet. One must look for:

D. K. Gupta, *Microskin Grafting for Vitiligo*,
DOI: 10.1007/978-1-84882-605-2_11, © Springer Science + Business Media B.V. 2009

- One piece construction for 100% centricity.
- Rounded edges avoiding dangerous sharp corners.
- Diamond chips grade large enough to provide maximum abrasion.
- The various sizes used are: 17 × 14, 17 × 10, 17 × 8, 15 × 10, 17 × 6, 17 × 4, 17 × 2.5 mm

11.5 Dermabrasion Wire Brushes

A high-speed rotary wire brush is used to remove the top layer of the skin. Commonly used sizes of high-speed rotary wire brushes are: 17 × 3, 17 × 6, 17 × 9, and 17 × 12 mm

The choice of diamond fraise or wire brush[1] for superficial dermabrasion is a matter of personal preference. The mechanism of action for both the techniques appears to be the removal of the epidermis and minimal or practically no injury to dermis particularly, when you are preparing the recipient site for vitiligo.

The diamond fraise is a more exacting instrument and with the recent introduction of the extra-coarse grit diamond fraise, the instrument is as abrasive as the standard wire brush. The diamond fraise is more easily controlled by the less experienced surgeon and because of its availability in many different shapes, widths, and grits, it provides greater versatility to the surgeon than the wire brush.

11.6 Dermabrasion Procedure

The areas to be treated are marked in sections and then prepared and draped in a sterile fashion. Three-point retraction is performed by using both hands of the surgical assistant and the surgeon's nondominant hand. The surgeon and staff should practice strict exposure precautions, including the wearing of protective face shields, to avoid contact with aerosolized matter and blood-borne pathogens.

The abrading instrument is properly held by placing the forefingers around the body of the instrument with the thumb outstretched on the shaft for stability and control. The results of dermabrasion depend on the coarseness of the abrading tip, the length of time the tip is applied to the skin, and the pressure used to apply the tip. Begin the abrasion in dependent areas, e.g., along the sides of the face, and work toward the center. This approach prevents bleeding from obscuring the skin to be abraded (Figs. 11.3–11.5).

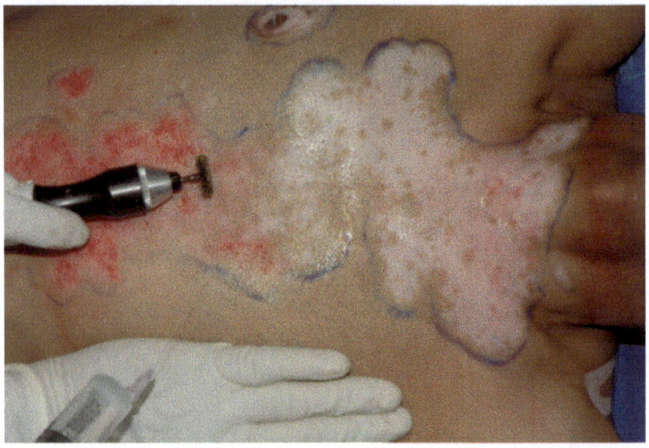

Fig. 11.3 Dermabrasion of extensive vitiliginous area with heavy duty electric hand engine. This quickly finishes the dermabrasion of large area within minutes

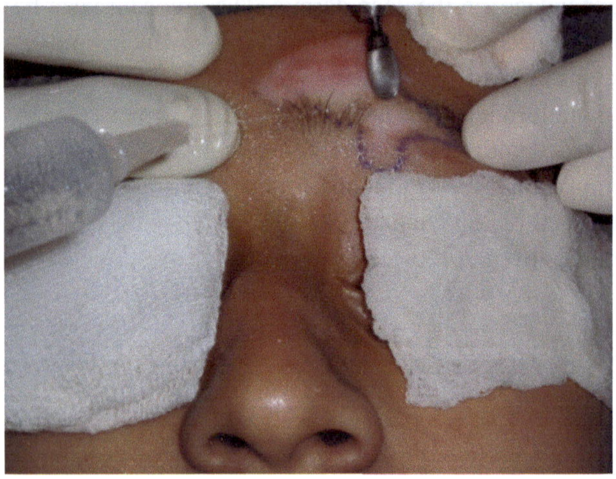

Fig. 11.4 Tungsten carbide serrated wheels used in small lesions for dermabrasion (serrated wheels are not commonly used)

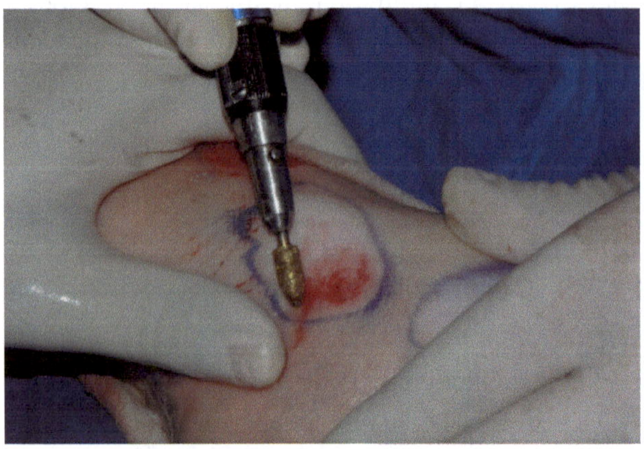

Fig. 11.5 Diamond fraise in use for superficial dermabrasion

The key to successful dermabrasion is controlling the wound created. The rotating head should be kept parallel to the skin surface, and the hand piece should be in motion at all the times. Begin by planing the epidermis down to the dermal junction. No bleeding occurs during dermabrasion through the epidermis because of the lack of blood vessels in this layer. Decreased pigmentation is encountered when the process continues through the epidermis. The dermoepidermal junction is reached next, followed by the papillary layer of the dermis. This layer is marked by uniform bleeding from punctate sites over a smooth, shiny surface. The deep papillary dermal layer is encountered when the surface becomes rough and when bleeding points increase.

At the periphery of the abraded area, lightly feather the borders by decreasing the pressure and the number of strokes to yield a uniform appearance. Exercise caution over bony prominences, where excessively deep dermabrasion commonly occurs.

Saline-moistened sponges can be applied to the treated area for 5–10 minutes to provide hemostasis.

11.7 Complications of Dermabrasion

Hypertrophic scarring is the most worrisome complication and results from dermabrasion through the deep dermis or an exaggerated inflammatory response (e.g., keloid formation). Persistent erythema and delayed reepithelialization should alert the physician and patient that scarring is imminent. Wounds that demonstrate a lack of reepithelialization by day 14 are at risk for hypertrophic scarring.

Infectious complications are unusual, but must be recognized quickly to prevent undesirable scarring. Postoperative viral infections, especially those due to herpes simplex virus, may occur despite prophylaxis. If pain, erythema, or ulcerations appear 7–10 days after the procedure, viral infection should be suspected, and a full-strength antiviral therapy should be administered. Infections due to staphylococcal, streptococcal, pseudomonal, or candidal bacteria may occur. If they do, wound cultures should be ordered, and appropriate oral or topical antibiotics or antifungal treatment should be started.

Milia, or intraepidermal collections of keratinaceous debris, are commonly observed after dermabrasion. These collections appear as small, white cysts.

Reference

1. Nelson BR, et al. A comparison of wire brush and diamond fraise superficial dermabrasion for photoaged skin. *J Am Acad Dermatol*. 1996;34:235–243.

Donor Area Selection

12

You can take skin from any of the convex surfaces of a patient's body, but the most convenient places are the fronts of the thighs. An appropriate donor site, typically the lateral, anterior or posterior part of the thigh, buttocks, or the medial aspect of the arm is selected. The skin here is easy to prepare, and easy to dress. If hip and knee are bent, you can also take the skin from the back of the thigh. For extensive vitiliginous area, a large flat donor surface is ideal for harvesting split thickness skin graft (STSG). The selection of the donor site should account for the size of the graft to be harvested, ability to hide the donor site under clothing, and ease of access to the area for follow-up care. The donor sites are usually cosmetically non important sites like the thighs, the buttocks or the waist (Figs. 12.1–12.7).

Other areas:

1. The cellular suspension is obtained from samples of skin of the hairy scalp after trypsinization.
2. Small pieces of uninvolved skin (2 × 1 cm) are taken for cultivation from a pudendal or axillary area.

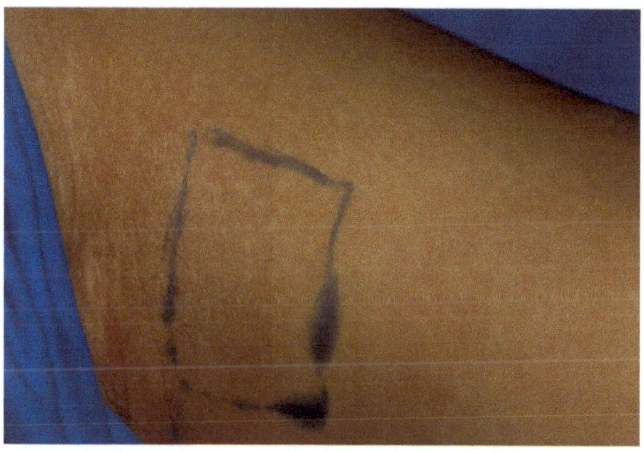

Fig. 12.1 Donor area: medial aspect of the upper arm

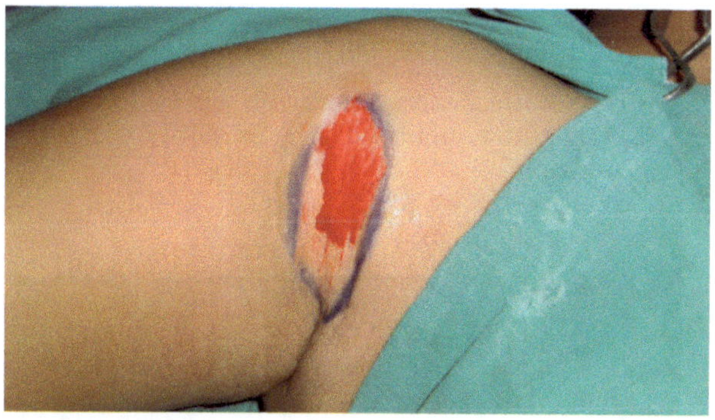

Fig. 12.2 Donor area: anterior axillary fold

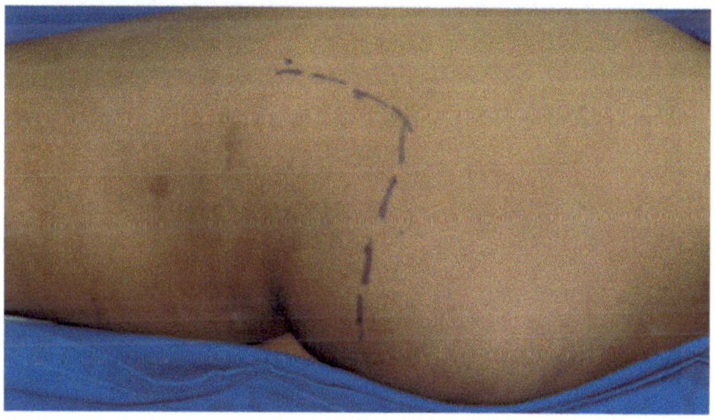

Fig. 12.3 Donor area: gluteal fold

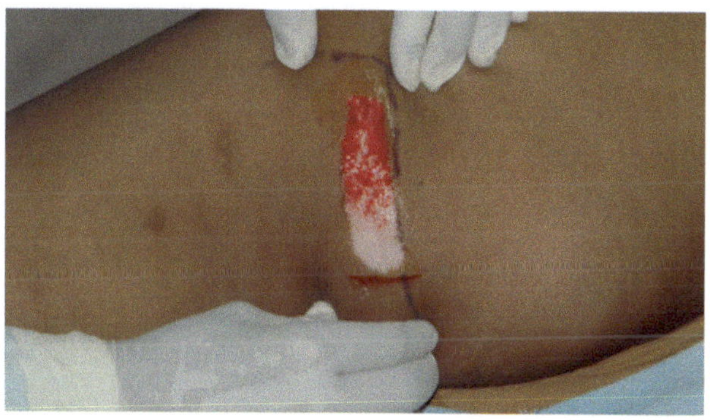

Fig. 12.4 Donor area: rawarea on gluteal fold following skin graft removal by Silver's knife

D. K. Gupta, *Microskin Grafting for Vitiligo*,
DOI: 10.1007/978-1-84882-605-2_12, © Springer Science + Business Media B.V. 2009

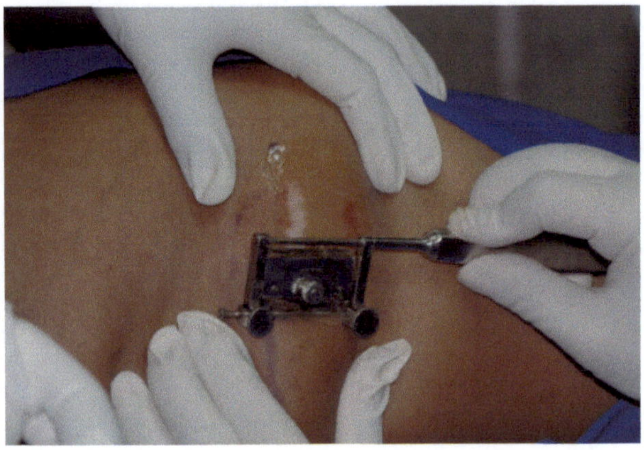

Fig. 12.5 Donor area: a very thin and narrow strip of skin graft can be removed from gluteal fold with the help of Silver's skin grafting knife. Donor area defect practically remains invisible in the fold. This narrow strip is sufficient for small to moderate vitiliginous area

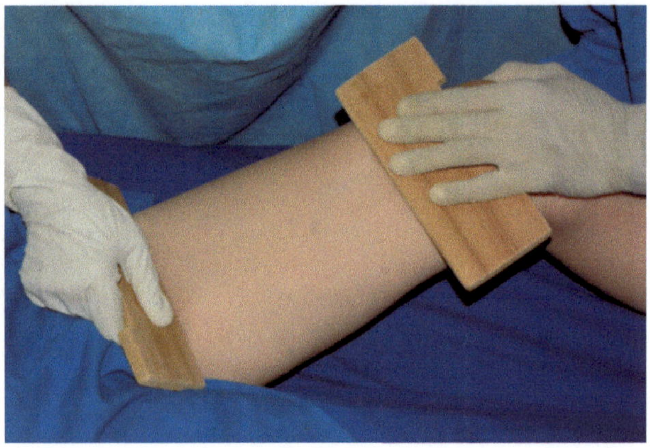

Fig. 12.7 Donor area: extensive graft can be removed from the anterior, lateral, medial and posterior aspect of the thigh

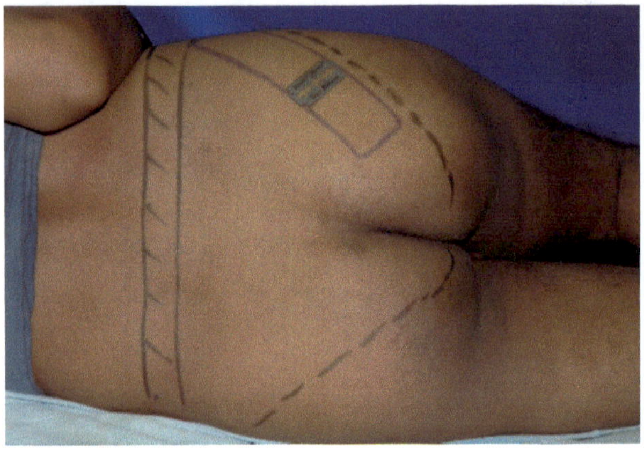

Fig. 12.6 Donor area: skin graft can be harvested from the gluteal region which remains covered by undergarments. Because of convexity of the buttocks, the graft can be removed with the help of power dermatome or Silver's knife

12.1 Donor Site Preparation

It is shaved, cleaned with soap and water, 70% ethanol and painted with povidone iodine and finally washed with normal saline and draped. It is anesthetized with the use of eutectic mixture of anesthetics (EMLA), infiltration anesthesia, nerve blocks or regional anesthesia. In extensive vitiligo, general anesthesia may be needed. The skin is stretched and thin or preferably ultra thin split thickness graft is obtained with Silver's skin grafting knife, Humby knife or powered dermatome. The superficial wound is then dressed with tulle gras.

Skin Graft Harvesting

13

13.1 Skin Harvesting Tools

A *dermatome* is a surgical instrument used to produce thin slices of skin from a donor area, in order to use them for making skin grafts. One of its main applications is for reconstituting skin areas damaged by grade 3 burns or trauma.

Dermatomes can be operated either manually or electrically. The first drum dermatomes, developed in the 1930s, were manually operated. Afterwards, dermatomes which were operated by air pressure, such as the Brown dermatome, achieved higher speed and precision. Electrical dermatomes are better for cutting out thinner and longer strips of skin with a more homogeneous thickness. Skin graft harvesting can be done by one of the following tools:

1. Free-hand knives
2. Various types of dermatomes
   - Knives
   - Drum
   - Powered (Electric or air)

13.1.1 Free-Hand Knives

These are manual dermatomes and the term knife or scalpel is used to describe them. Their disadvantages are harvesting of grafts with irregular edges and grafts of variable thickness. The operator has to be experienced in their use for optimal results.

13.1.2 Types of Dermatomes

There are several types of dermatomes, usually named after their inventor (Fig. 13.1).

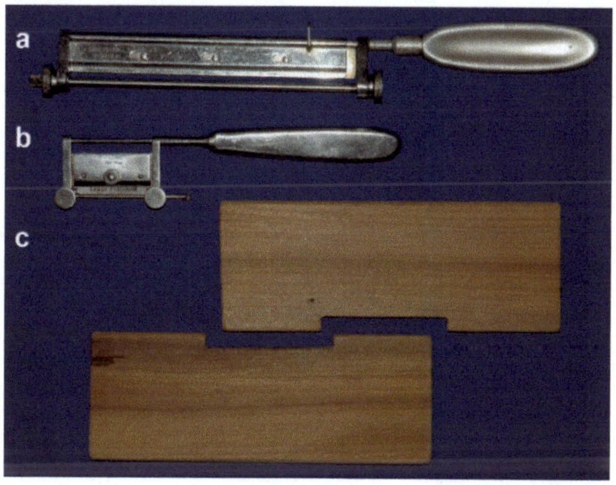

Fig. 13.1 The standard equipments for skin grafting. (**a**) Watson's modification of Humby knife. Most popular and useful skin grafting tool for harvesting different thickness of wide skin graft. (**b**) Silver's skin graft knife. Stainless double edged razor blades are used for taking small grafts. Its disadvantage is that it can only cut narrow strips of skin. (**c**) A pair of soft wooden Board with rounded edges

13.1.2.1 Knives

- Silver's miniature knife, ideal for the harvesting of small grafts.
- Sober hand dermatome
- Skin grafting with a modified safety razor is not yet made commercially, so you will have to make it by yourself.
- Watson modification of Humby knife: Sterilize only the knife, the blades are disposable and presterilized. Autoclaving will blunt them.

13.1.2.2 Drum Dermatome

- Padgett dermatome, was the first rotary drum manual dermatome to be devised.

D. K. Gupta, *Microskin Grafting for Vitiligo*,
DOI: 10.1007/978-1-84882-605-2_13, © Springer Science + Business Media B.V. 2009

13.1.2.3 Powered (Electric or Air) Dermatomes

- Battery-operated Davol dermatome
- Humeca Battery operated dermatome
- Padgett dermatome
- Zimmer air dermatome

The Davol dermatome lends itself well to use in office-based surgery; it has a disposable head, a preset width, and a rechargeable battery, although the thickness of the graft to be harvested is operator dependent. The Padgett dermatome allows the surgeon to adjust the graft thickness and width. Despite the fact that both the Padgett and Davol dermatomes reliably produce STSGs of even thickness, the quality of the graft has been described as highly technique dependent. The Zimmer air dermatome tends to be less technique dependent in harvesting STSGs of predetermined uniform width and thickness.

In co-operation with the Dutch surgeon Dr. Willem Nugteren, Humeca developed a new dermatome for freehanded harvesting of a 30-mm (1¼ in.) wide split skin graft with a predetermined thickness of about 0.25 mm (0.01 in.). The dermatome is held firmly against the tautly held skin at a predetermined angle and a graft of the desired length is quickly cut. No lateral movements are required.

13.1.3 Silver's Skin Graft Knife Handle

"New" to the range, the Silver's stainless steel "miniature" skin graft knife was originally developed by H.L.Silver in Toronto, Canada. Combined with surgical stainless double edged razor blades, it is ideal for taking small intricate grafts from areas which would not be accessible with the larger standard knives. Although used mainly within Plastic, Reconstructive and Oral surgery, the Silver's can also be used for the debridement of wounds. It is $7^1/_2''$ long and uses a double-edge razor blade.

13.1.4 Sober Hand Dermatome

Skin graft cutting with a Sober hand dermatome is just like a graft cutting with modified safety razor dermatome. The ability to cut a split-thickness skin graft free-handedly, has been regarded as a skill acquired only by long experience. Several devices have been improvised to simplify this task. However, the size and elaborate arrangements of dermatomes often preclude their use, especially if the need is in an emergency room, a clinic or at the patient's bedside. Besides sophisticated dermatomes are costly and more adequate for harvesting larger skin grafts.

13.2 Grafting with a Modified Safety Razor

Skin grafting with a modified safety razor is not yet made commercially, so you will have to make it by yourself. One can convert the safety razor into a dermatome by removing the central strut on one side and placing another safety razor blade with its sharp edge that has been ground as a shim.

13.2.1 Humby Skin Grafting Knife

This is the most popular and commonly used skin grafting knife. With this, one can take broad and large skin graft quickly. The disadvantage of this usual dermatome blade is its length which makes many areas inaccessible to operation with such a blade. This is especially so in children, the convexity of whose limbs allows grafts, often only an inch wide. We have in fact, found that with the narrow dermatome (modified safety razor, Sober hand dermatome) we can take skin from practically anywhere on the body. The narrow strips of appropriate thickness is taken in such a way that the donor area heals so quickly that they may give new grafts, if necessary, within 3 weeks. One blade is sufficient for any but the very largest grafts. The simplicity of the narrow dermatome machine is such that skin grafting can be done by every surgeon or general practitioner.

13.2.2 Cutting Split Skin Grafts

You can slice the superficial part of some skin (a split skin graft) from another part of the patient's body (the donor area) and lay this on his wound (the recipient site).

It will probably, "take" (live). The donor site will heal, because the whole of his epidermis can regenerate from the deeper parts of his sweat glands and hair follicles which you have left behind.

You can cut split skin grafts thinner or thicker by varying the setting of the knife. A thinner split skin graft: (1) resists infection better, (2) takes more easily, (3) allows the donor area to recover quickly.

13.2.3 Preoperative Details

No specific preoperative evaluation is unique to skin grafting.

As with all dermatologic surgery, thorough preoperative history taking is critical; the history should include information about the patient's medications (particularly those with anticoagulant properties), allergies, bleeding diatheses, frequent or recurrent infections, and general wound healing.

Other preoperative considerations include the potential for postoperative trauma to the area caused by patient activities (particularly those involving shearing forces), the patient's ability to care for the wounds (at both the donor and recipient sites), and the surgeon's assessment of the patient's expectations.

13.3 Preoperative Preparation

Bathe the patient. Shave the donor site and scrub it well with soap and water and then swab it with mild antiseptic solution such as cetrimide.

13.4 Equipment

A skin grafting knife, two graft boards, liquid paraffin, skin hooks, nontoothed forceps for handling the graft, vaseline gauze, a bowl of sterile saline to put the graft in, sterile cotton wool, and a sterile screw topped jar for storing excess graft and two trained assistants (Figs. 13.1 and 13.2).

13.5 Anesthesia for Skin Grafting

If possible, use local anesthesia for the donor area, so that he is more likely to cooperate. (1) Use plenty of very dilute local anesthetic, such as 0.4% lignocaine with adrenaline, to puff out the skin all over the donor site. If you raise it like a plateau, it will be easier to cut.

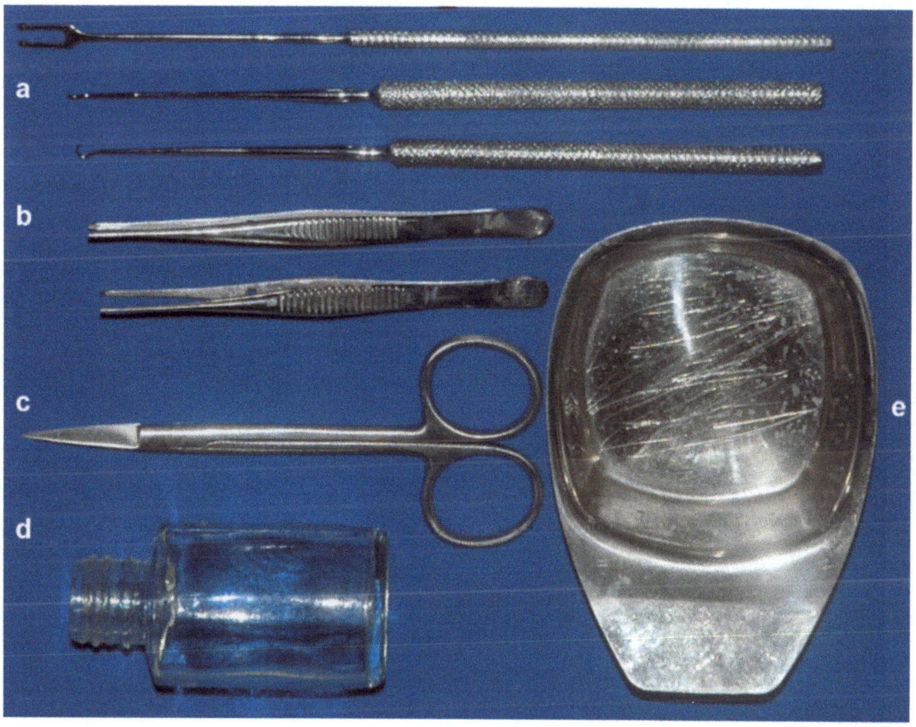

Fig. 13.2 Additional skin grafting tools. (**a**) Skin hooks. (**b**) Tooth and non tooth dissecting forceps. (**c**) Scissors. (**d**) Glass container for storing skin graft at 4°C in refrigerator. (**e**) Stainless steel bowl

Raise blebs in suitable places and then infiltrate the whole area with a long needle just below the dermis, as in (Figs. 13.3–13.5). This is the best method of local

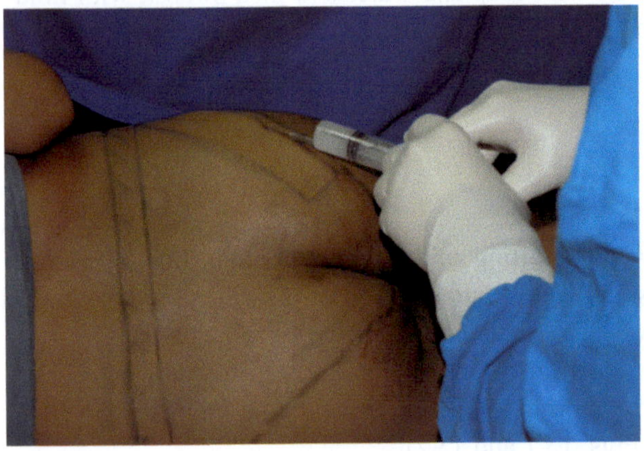

Fig. 13.3 After raising the subcutaneous blebs by using 30G needle in suitable places of gluteal region, infiltrate the whole area with a long needle just below the dermis

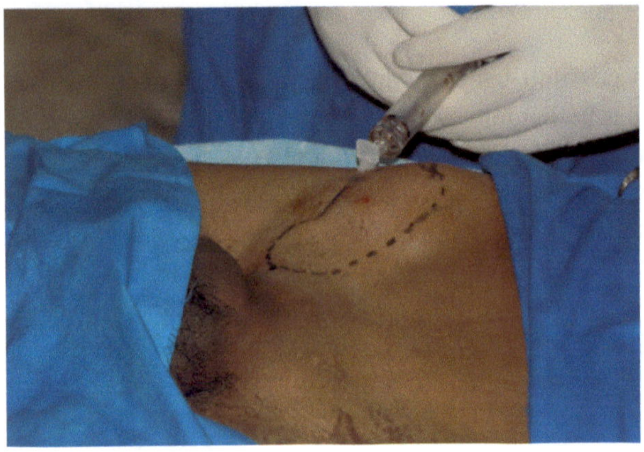

Fig. 13.4 Right groin as a donor site. Local infiltrative (0.4% lignocaine) anesthesia

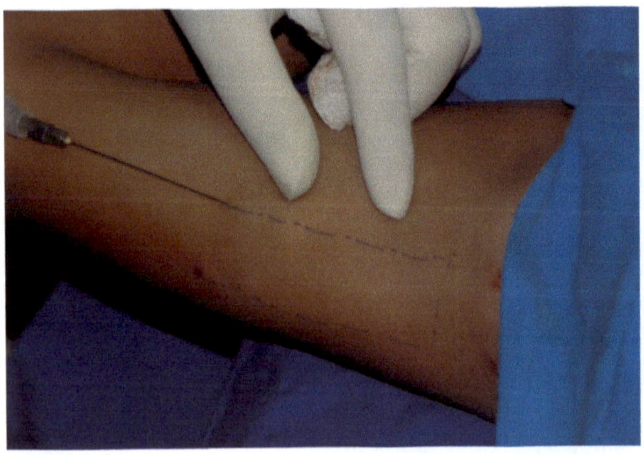

Fig. 13.5 Medial side of upper arm is being infiltrated with dilute local anesthetic solution

anesthesia for the arm. (2) Take skin from his thigh by blocking both his femoral nerve and the lateral cutaneous nerve of his thigh. (3) If you are going to take an extensive graft from several sites, give him a general anesthesia. (4) You can use ketamine; if you give him diazepam at the end of the operation, he is unlikely to thrash about as he recovers and so disturb the graft. (5) Eutectic mixture of local anesthetic (EMLA) is used for surface anesthesia for superficial dermabrasion and small graft harvesting.

13.5.1 Eutectic Mixture of Lidocaine and Prilocaine (EMLA)

EMLA® Cream (lidocaine and prilocaine cream) is an emulsion in which oil phase is a eutectic mixture of lidocaine and prilocaine in a ratio of 1:1 by weight. This eutectic mixture has a melting point below room temperature and therefore both local anesthetics exist as liquid oil rather than as crystals. EMLA® is indicated as a topical anesthetic for use on normal intact skin only. Cream is applied using a spatula to form a thick even layer of 2–3 mm. Leave Cream with occlusive dressing for minimum 1–2 h, as per the need, before surgery.

13.6 Positions for Cutting Grafts

It is essential to keep the donor area surface flat, taut and stretched, for smooth uniform thickness graft cutting. Various positions for smooth graft cutting is shown in figures (Figs. 13.6–13.8).

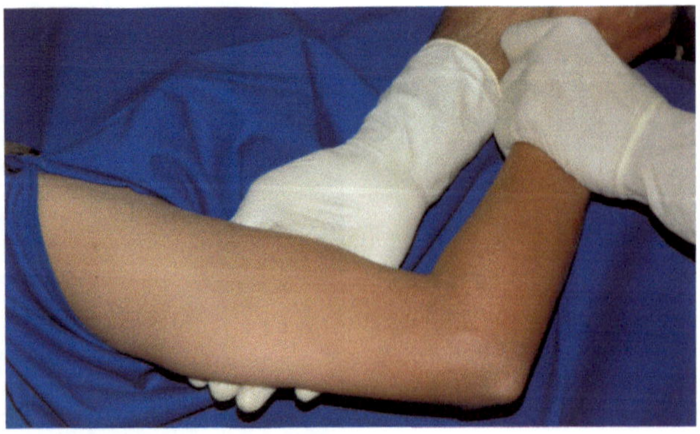

Fig. 13.6 Positioning the arm for cutting a split thickness skin graft

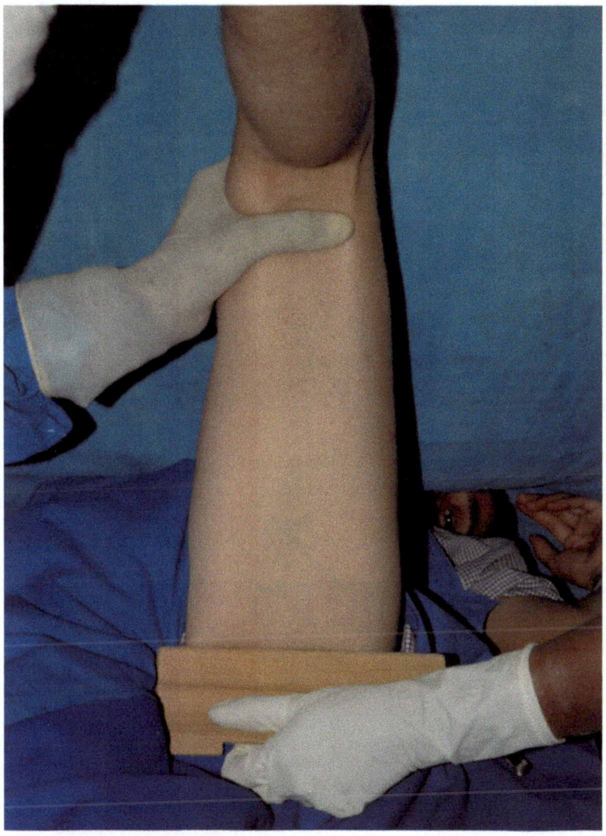

Fig. 13.7 Positioning the thigh for cutting a split thickness skin graft from posterior side of thigh and the way the surface is presented to provide the maximum area of flat skin.

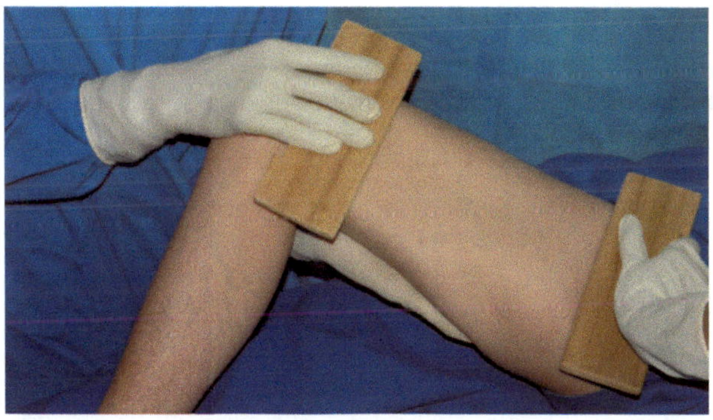

Fig. 13.8 Lateral side of thigh as good donor area

13.7 Cutting the Graft

Place yourself comfortably before starting. The leg on the patient's right side, and assuming you are right handed, cut from below upwards, with a forehand stroke. On his left side, cut from above downwards.

Ask your assistant to support the skin of the patient's thigh from underneath, so as to make its upper surface flat, and under slight tension from side to side. This will allow you to make a smooth cut with neater edges.

Abduct the patient's arm, and place it on a wide arm rest or table. Ask your assistant to put one of his gloved hands behind it, so as to stretch and flatten the skin on its antero-medial surface. Cut from his shoulder downwards.

Stand inside his abducted right arm, or outside his abducted left arm.

The skin of the upper arm is thin, so don't cut a full thickness graft inadvertently.

In Humby knife, the thickness of the skin to be cut is controlled by a rod. The position of this rod is controlled by a screw at one end, and a graduated lock nut at the other. You will have to learn by practice, what thickness of graft these calibrations represent. Hold the knife up to the light and vary the distance between the blade and the rod (Fig. 13.9). If you think you could just slip a razor blade between them (a little less than 0.5 mm), one should keep it little narrow for thin graft. You can take the help of feeler gauges. Make it too narrow rather than too wide, because if the graft is too thin, you can always thicken it. If the rod touches the blade anywhere they are far too close. Make sure the blade and the knife are flexible, so the thickness of the graft also depends on how hard you press. After the selection of the appropriate device, the donor site is lubricated with sterile sodium chloride solution or mineral oil. Lubricate the back of the knife with liquid

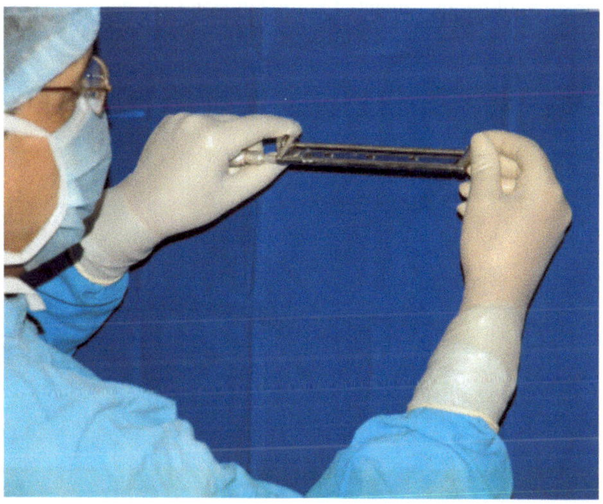

Fig. 13.9 Hold the knife up to the light. Looking at the gap between the roller and the blade to adjust the thickness and the cut

paraffin. Keep it clear of the roller, or it may cause the graft to wind round it.

Ask your assistant to hold one board behind the knife, to keep the board still, and to press on the skin so as to hold it flat and in tension, as you move the knife. Use the second board in your left hand to keep the skin flattened in front of the advancing knife blade. Advance the board and the blade together along the limb. Apply the knife to the skin at a slight angle and use a regular sawing movement. Advance it slowly, and press gently. The graft usually collects in folds on the knife. If it does not, ask your assistant to pick its end up. When you get to the end of the graft, either cut it with scissors, or bring the knife to the surface. The movement of the dermatome in the surgeon's hand has been likened to a plane's landing and taking off. The newly harvested graft is placed in sterile sodium chloride solution (Figs. 13.10–13.16).

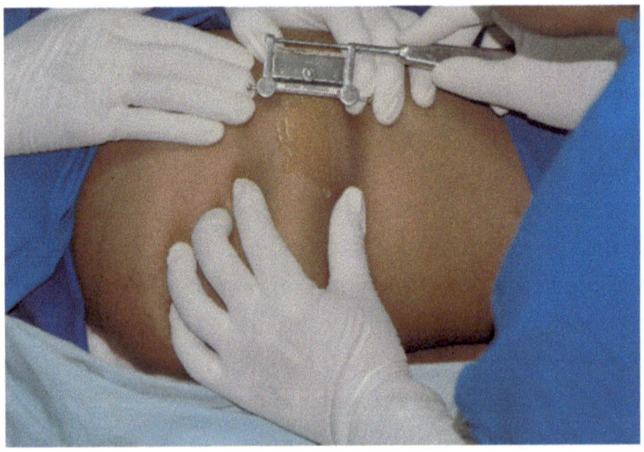

Fig. 13.10 Skin is being cut from the gluteal fold with the help of Silver's knife. Assistant stretches the skin in the opposite direction of the movement of knife. Surgeon's left hand pinches the skin of gluteal crease so that skin is lifted up as shown

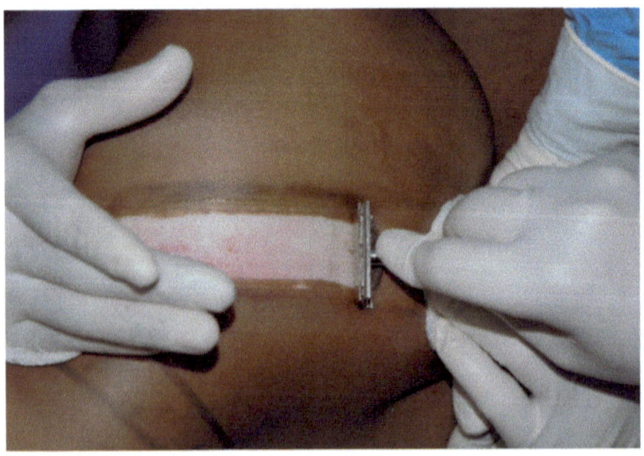

Fig. 13.11 Graft is being cut from the tautly held skin of the gluteal region with the help of hand dermatome by its dragging action. No lateral movements are required

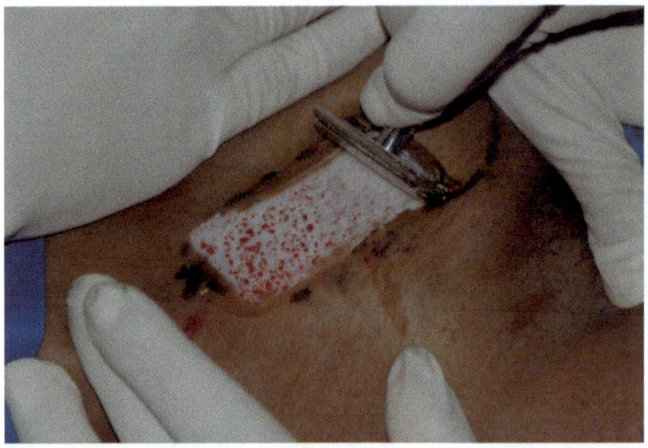

Fig. 13.12 Split thickness skin graft (STSG) removal from the groin by Modified razor dermatome

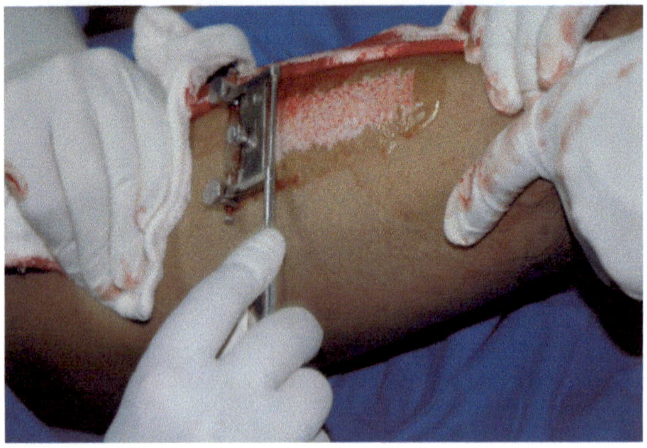

Fig. 13.13 Graft is being cut from the anterolateral side of the thigh with the help of Silver's knife. Assistant stretches the skin behind the knife towards the direction of knee

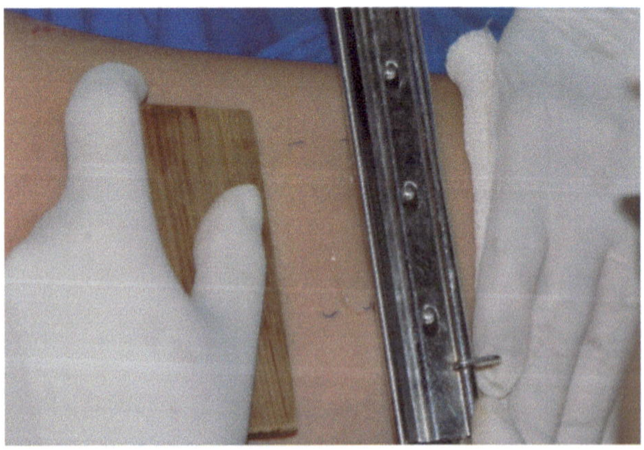

Fig. 13.14 Graft cutting from thigh. Assistant keeps the skin taut. Surgeon's left hand stretches the skin in the direction of forward movement of knife and keeps it flat by moving the wooden board in synchronization with knife's movement

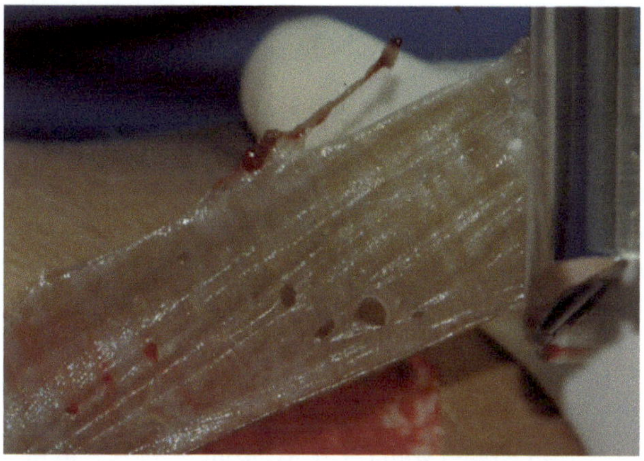

Fig. 13.15 Ultra thin Split thickness skin graft (STSG-UT): nearly epidermal thick ultra thin graft removed from the thigh. One can notice the transparency of ultra thin graft. It is practically a sort of blister epidermal graft

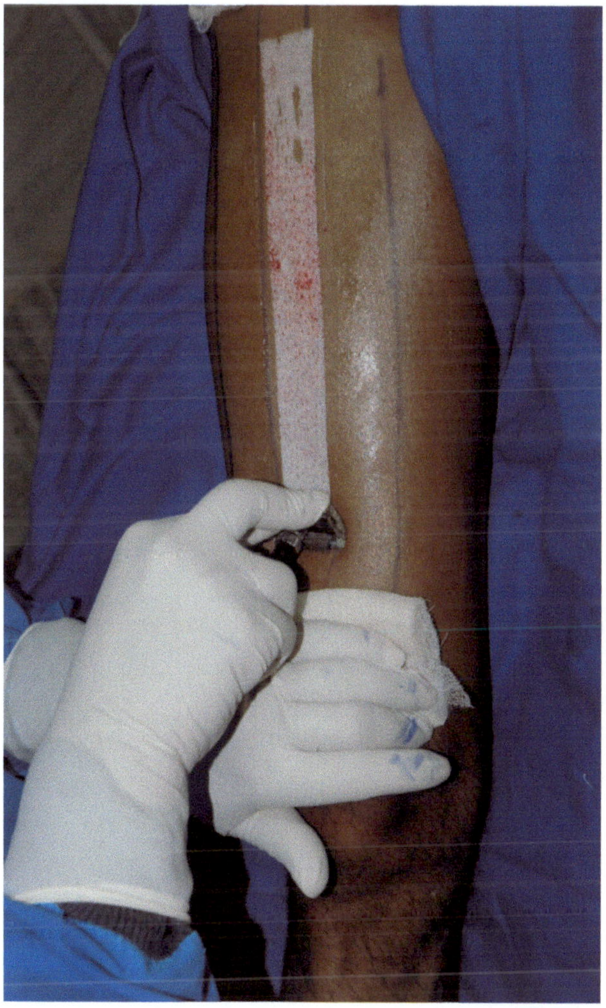

Fig. 13.16 Thin split thickness skin graft (STSG-T) cutting from thigh. Thin graft removed from the anterior aspect of the thigh by using modified razor hand dermatome

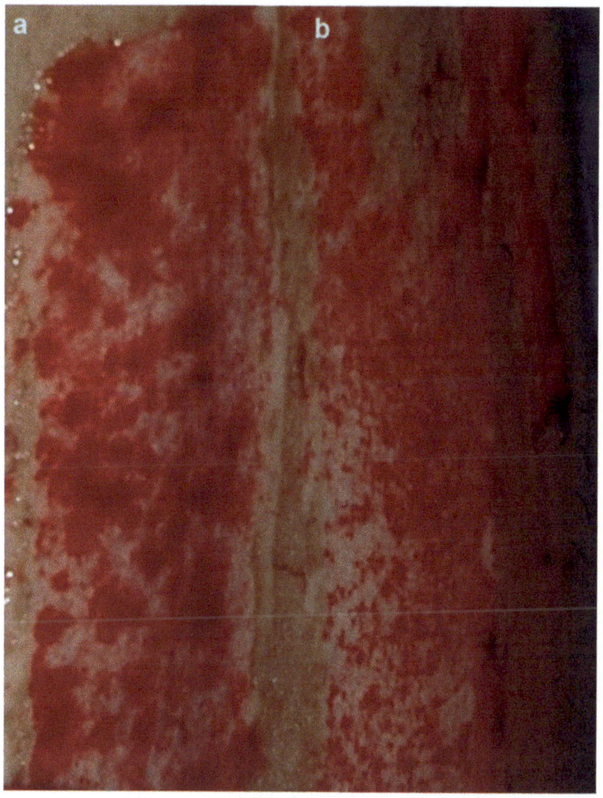

Fig. 13.17 Pattern of bleeding points in the donor area. (**a**) Large bleeding point from thicker graft. (**b**) Tiny bleeding points from thinner ones

CAUTION! (1) Don't force the knife down the limb. (2) Don't stop or pull the knife backwards. (2) You will be wise to take more graft than you need and store it, so that you can apply it later to areas which do not take.

After you have cut about 1 cm of graft, inspect it for thickness. Assess it by: (1) Translucency; a very thin graft is translucent, like tissue paper. Thicker grafts are progressively more opaque. (2) The pattern of bleeding points; a thin graft produces many tiny points, a thicker graft fewer larger ones (Fig. 13.17).

Keep the graft covered with saline soaked swabs until you are ready to store or apply it.

13.7.1 Graft Take

The harvested skin graft is completely separated from its vascular supply prior to its transplantation in the recipient site. The graft proceeds through several physiologic stages before the newly transplanted tissue is assimilated (i.e., "takes").

The initial stage of graft healing, termed plasmatic imbibition, occurs within the first 24–48 hours after the placement of the graft on the recipient bed. During this process, the donor tissues receive their nutrition through the absorption of plasma from the recipient wound bed via capillary action. In this phase of healing, the graft is white and may appear somewhat edematous. Furthermore, because nutrients can be absorbed more effectively over shorter distances, thinner grafts tend to survive better in this stage of graft healing. In addition, during this phase of healing, a fibrin network is created between the graft and the recipient bed. The recipient bed then generates vascular buds that grow into the fibrin network.

After imbibition, is the phase of graft healing termed inosculation. This phase starts 48–72 hours after grafting and may continue for as long as 1 week after grafting. During this time, the aforementioned vascular buds anastomose with both preexisting and newly formed vessels. This revascularization of the skin graft, which occurs more rapidly in an STSG than in an FTSG, is initially accompanied by a mottled appearance, and then a vascular erythematous blush or, occasionally, a slightly cyanotic appearance. In most recipient areas, revascularization occurs from both the base and the periphery of the recipient bed during this process.

Lymphatics develop in the graft tissue at approximately 1 week after transplantation, and reinnervation of the graft may begin as early as the first few weeks, although many grafts may have some degree of permanent anesthesia. A unique phenomenon of vascular bridging has been described to account for revascularization in relatively avascular recipient beds. In this phenomenon, vascular ingrowths occur from the relatively, highly vascularized lateral aspects of the recipient bed and bridges across the avascular base of the recipient bed. However, for vascular bridging to occur, the recipient area must remain small, and the area that immediately surrounds the graft must be highly vascularized.

13.8 The Donor Site Care

Minimize blood oozing by immediately applying a moist pressure pack. Later remove the pack and replace it by vaseline gauze, and a pressure bandage. Pad the wound generously to prevent blood soaking through, and bandage it, preferably with an elastic bandage. At 9–11 days remove the dressings. If the dressings have stuck to the donor site, leave them in place. If you tear them off, the wound will be very slow to heal. If the donor site become infected, treat it like any other superficial wound with frequent cleaning and changing of dressings.

13.9 Postoperative Care for Skin Grafts

If a joint has to be grafted, a splint over the dressings is very useful.

Leave the dressing for 7–9 days, unless there is some good reason for looking at it. Do the first dressing yourself, so that you can inspect your handiwork. First remove only the superficial layers. Leave the layer of vaseline gauze which was used to spread the split skin. Remove this later when the graft is firmly adherent.

13.9.1 Storing Grafts

You can store a graft in an ordinary refrigerator at 4°C. Put the graft in a sterile screw capped bottle labeled with the patient's name and the date of graft harvesting. The sooner you apply it the better. It may be wise to discard grafts after 8 days, although it may be kept for 2 or 3 weeks.

14 Microskin Grafting Tools

Apart from standard skin graft harvesting tools, you will need two more things. One is a spraying device for spreading the microskin grafts and the second is a stainless steel sieve and a shallow tray for filtration and collection of normal saline following spraying or floatation of microskin grafts on muslin sheets (Figs. 14.1 and 14.2).

14.1 Muslin Tulle Gras

For microskin grafts, it is best to make vaselined gauze (tulle gras) using muslin (fine woven fabric) for spreading and dressing. Muslin is cut in rectangles of 10 × 10 cm, packing them firmly in a metal (aluminium) box, and then impregnating with hot Vaseline, the level of which should reach the uppermost layer of muslin.

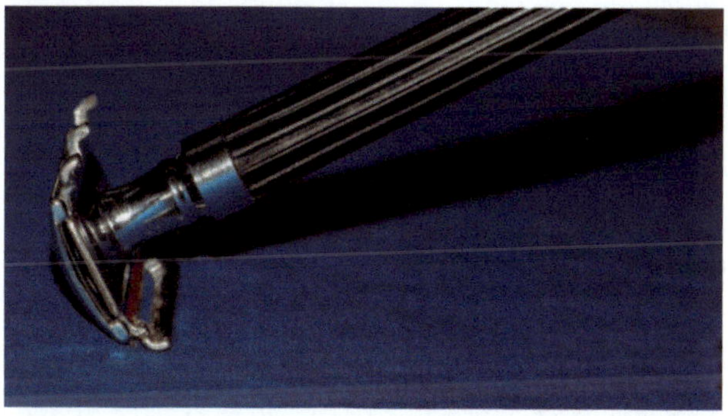

Fig. 14.2 Modified safety razor dermatome

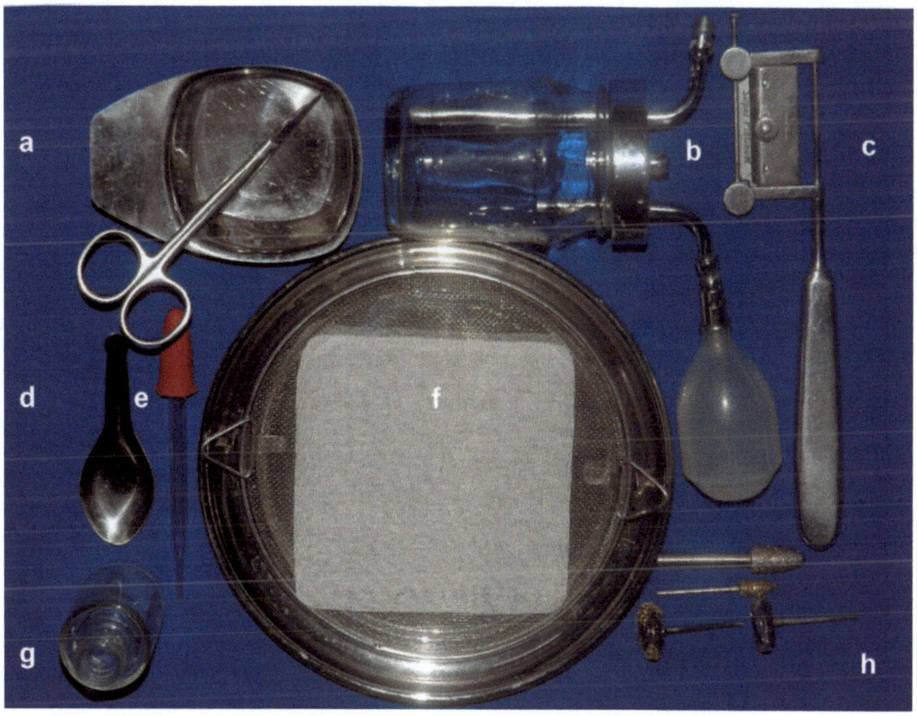

Fig. 14.1 (**a**) Stainless steel bowl and scissors; (**b**) spraying device; (**c**) silver's skin grafting knife; (**d**) spoon for floatation and spreading of MSGs; (**e**) dropper; (**f**) shallow stainless steel tray, sieve and muslin piece; (**g**) glass container for graft storage; (**h**) diamond fraises and wire brushes

D. K. Gupta, *Microskin Grafting for Vitiligo*,
DOI: 10.1007/978-1-84882-605-2_14,

Complete impregnation and sterilization may then be achieved by heating the entire vessel at 140–150°C for an hour.

This technique, with the use of muslin, makes a very fine-meshed tulle, which is easy to cut into small squares and more adaptable in shape, and is particularly suitable for small vitiliginous areas (Figs. 14.3–14.6).

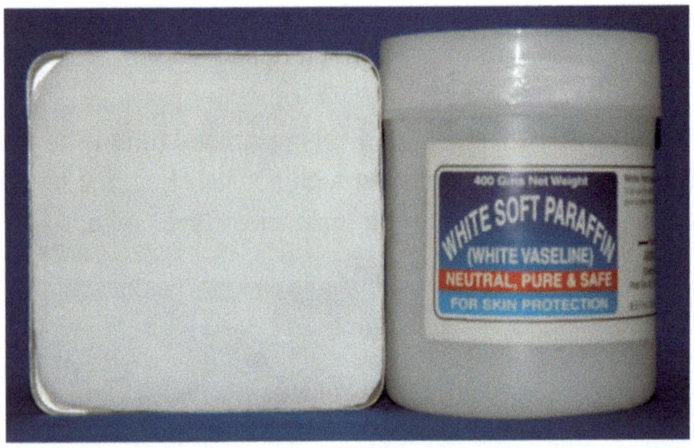

Fig. 14.3 Muslin cut sheets in aluminium square box (10 × 10 cm) and white soft paraffin

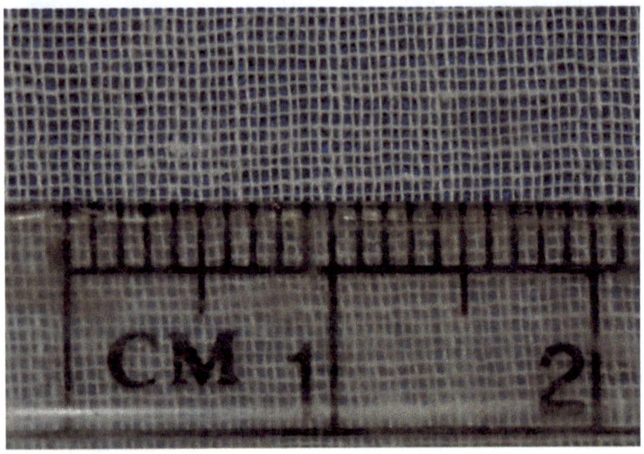

Fig. 14.4 The width of three interstices of muslin sheet equal to 1 mm

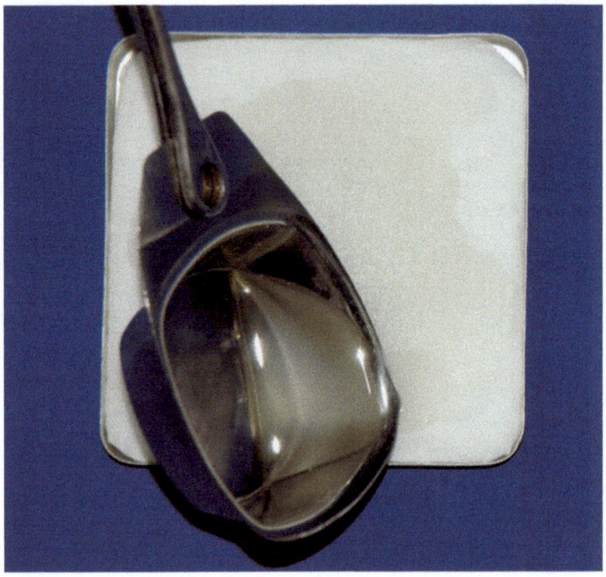

Fig. 14.5 Melted warm white soft paraffin spilled over the muslin kept in aluminum box

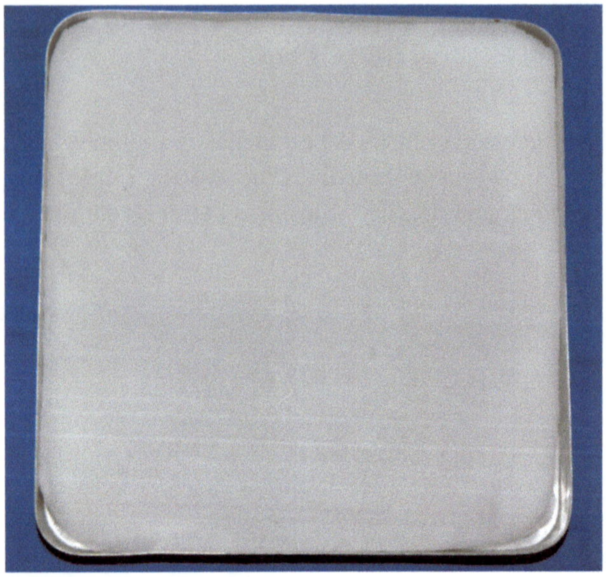

Fig. 14.6 Sterilized ready to use vaselined muslin tulle gras. Muslin is just saturated with white soft paraffin

Techniques of Microskin Grafts Distribution on Ablated Vitiliginous Areas 15

15.1 Microskin Grafting for Repigmentation of Vitiligo by Direct Spread Method

Microskin grafts (MSGs) are prepared by mincing the ultra thin or thin split thickness skin graft (STSG-UT, STSG-T) with scissors into tiny pieces smaller than 1 mm in size. These MSGs are then evenly spread on the abraded vitiliginous area with the help of forceps or spatula. The grafting operation must be performed gently and carefully, avoiding excessive movement of the MSGs on the wound. The wound is wrapped with petrolatum gauze, cotton pads and splinted, in order to keep the recipient site immobile near joint.

The recipient site is examined 7–11 days postoperatively. The MSGs that do not vascularize on recipient area due to its non contact on recipient bed become black and falls out as crust. This again emphasizes the usefulness of very thin and even spread of MSGs on recipient site and at the same time minimizes the donor area.

The direct spread method is quite useful in limited vitiliginous areas like focal and segmental stable vitiligo. Here, the expansion ratio of donor to recipient area is about 1:1.

I used to apply MSGs by direct spread method with the help of a spatula in few of my earlier cases of vitiligo. In direct spread method, much more donor area is needed as compared to other methods of distribution. Direct spread method is thus useful only in small stable vitiligo and not in extensive ones (Figs. 15.1-15.4).

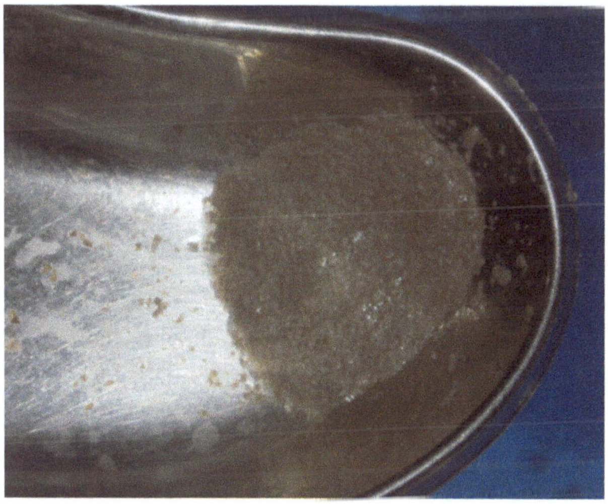

Fig. 15.1 Prepared microskin grafts (MSGs) with the help of scissor

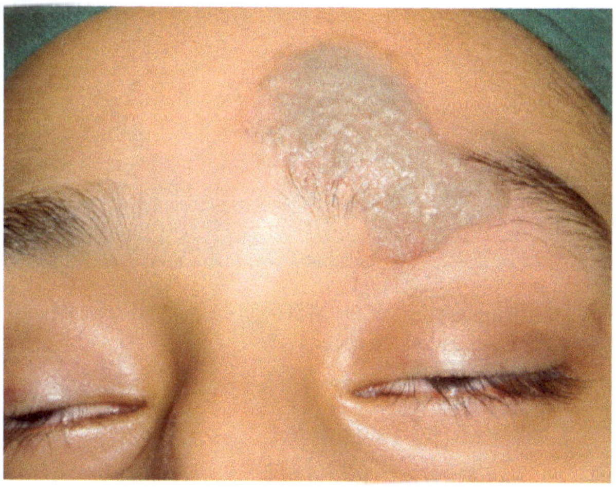

Fig. 15.2 Direct spread of the MSGs on the forehead with the help of the tip and the back of small dissecting forceps (MSGs made from ultra thin STSG)

D. K. Gupta, *Microskin Grafting for Vitiligo*,
DOI: 10.1007/978-1-84882-605-2_15, © Springer Science + Business Media B.V. 2009

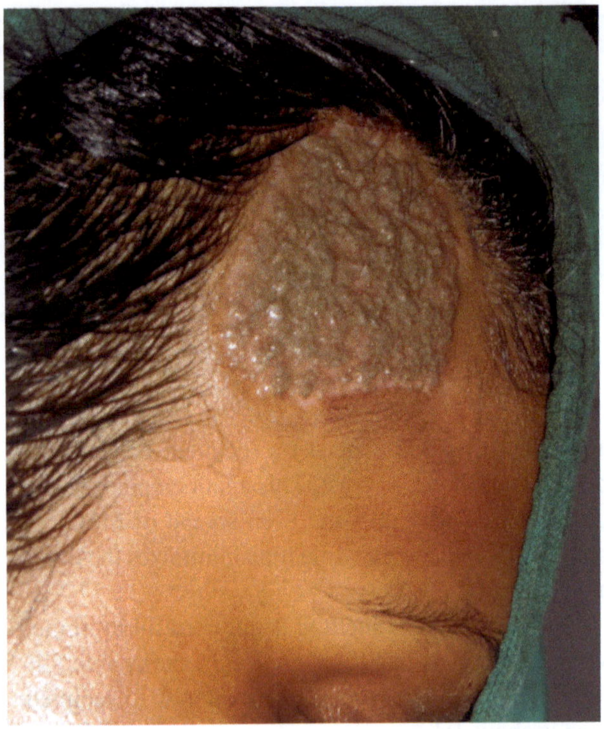

Fig. 15.3 Direct spread of the MSGs on the forehead (MSGs made from thin STSG)

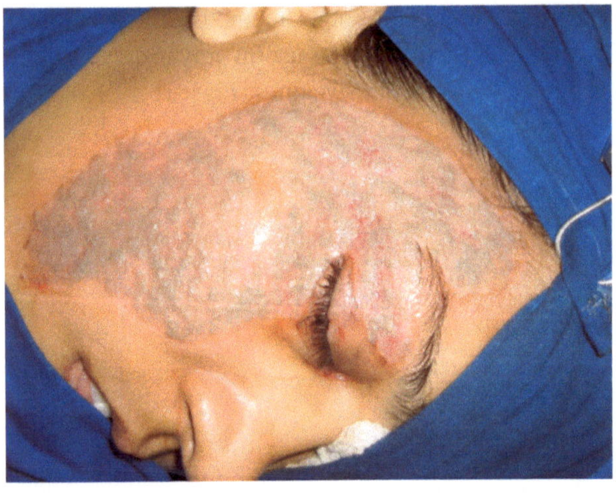

Fig. 15.4 Direct spread of the MSGs on dermabraded post burn dyschromia present on the cheek

15.2 Microskin Grafting by Floatation Method

The technique of transplantation of autologous microskin grafts (MSGs) is used in the treatment of vitiligo patients. Preparation of MSGs includes: (1) mincing of split-thickness skin autografts into skin particles (SPs) with the help of scissor; (2) dispersing the SPs evenly on a piece of muslin cloth by a spoon; (3) transferring the SPs to the abraded surface of vitiliginous area; (4) Superficial dermabrasion followed immediately by MSG applications are performed on body sites, including extremities, chest and abdomen, back, face and neck. Advantages of this technique are: (1) the great potential of the MSG to provide a large expansion ratio of 1:3–1:10. (2) Ease of preparation and application with low cost, compared to cultured epidermal sheet grafts. (3) Economical use of autografts. (4) The procedure is simple. (5) Less scar or no scar formation on donor area as the graft removed were thin or ultra thin in nature. (6) There are no scars on the recipient site. This new technique is effective, simple and feasible in extensive vitiligo.

The large vitiliginous area may be difficult to repigment with split thickness autologous skin sheet graft. On the other hand, split thickness skin graft may be used as a microskin graft after the mincing process, which reduces the size of the MSGs less than 1 mm.

A piece of ultra thin or thin split thickness skin graft (0.15–0.30 mm in thickness) is harvested from the patient and minced with scissor into tiny pieces smaller than 1 mm and then immersed in normal saline. The minced skin gradually starts floating on the surface of the normal saline. The floating particles of skin are removed from the saline and evenly spread on the muslin cloth with a spoon. The muslin cloth is turned over carefully, leaving the micrografts in contact with the abraded vitiliginous area of the patient.

One can cut the muslin sheet (that carries MSGs) into pieces and then apply it according to the size of vitiliginous areas.

The recipient area was bandaged gently and carefully, avoiding excessive shearing movement. The area near the joint must be splinted to avoid dislodgement and migration of the MSGs.

The survival of micrografts is related to their contact positioning, the preferred orientation is one when the dermis of the microskin grafts is in contact with the wound. As many pieces of the microskin grafts are an irregular polyhedron in shape, they can make contact with the wound in three ways:

(1) Upward direction, epithelial side up; (2) lateral direction, epithelial side laterally; (3) downward direction, epithelial side down.

There is no problem of survival when the microskin grafts are in an upward direction. When the microskin grafts are orientated in a lateral or downward direction, they first develop epidermal cysts or epidermal columns, then extend upwards to cover the surface of the wound or meet with the epidermal layer from other micrografts. The microskin grafts orientated in a non-upward direction can survive because they are very small and are surrounded by microlacerated vitiliginous area abraded by rotatory wire brush or large particle diamond fraise; therefore, they can be supplied with blood from any direction, but spread of pigmentation from such grafts are slow and less as compared to normally oriented graft.

The microskin grafts should be as small as possible. The smaller the size of the micrograft, the larger their number, so that the autografts can be utilized more extensively. The ratio of donor site to recipient site surface area is 1:3, to a maximum of upto 1:10 by floatation method. The vitiliginous areas get pigmented completely in 3–6 months time. With very extensive vitiligo, this ratio can be up to 1:15 or more, but would take a long time to repigment and may even need secondary microskin grafting for residual vitiliginous patches.

The newer cellular graft techniques like keratinocytes and melanocytes suspension can extend the donor to recipient area ratio upto 1:10 and are helpful to cover the large vitiliginous area in a single sitting but at the cost of a good laboratory and infrastructure. The microskin grafting may be considered to be similar to cultured epithelium in certain respects, the skin in the former is cultured in vivo, and the skin in the later is cultured in vitro. On the other hand, however, cultured skin cells in vitro require sophisticated equipment, and it takes 3–4 weeks to grow a thin layer of epithelium. The microskin grafts are cultured in vivo and the wound provides the most suitable conditions (i.e., temperature, moisture, oxygen, nutrition, etc.) for skin cell growth. This procedure of microskin grafting neither needs a complex culture process nor does it require a long time for culture in vitro.

Attention should be paid to the following points during microskin grafting: split thickness autografts of size less than 0.30 mm thickness are the best. If the autografts are thicker, the minced skin tends to form small balls with the epithelial side outwards and thus can not survive on the wound (Fig. 15.28). Theoretically, microskin grafts orientated upwards (epithelial side up) take best. They fuse together better than those in other direction; in these areas, the surface of the pigmented healed wound may be smoother.

I have practically seen that if the microskin grafts are prepared from the thin (<0.30 mm) split thickness skin graft, the results are excellent. The digital image analysis of these microskin grafts on the recipient bed showed mixed pattern of orientation e.g., both upward and downward direction of the grafts. In spite of this, uniform pigmentation is achieved at vitiliginous area in less than 3–4 months time. Greater the density of the microskin grafts on the vitiliginous area, lesser the time required for complete repigmentation (Fig. 15.5–15.7).

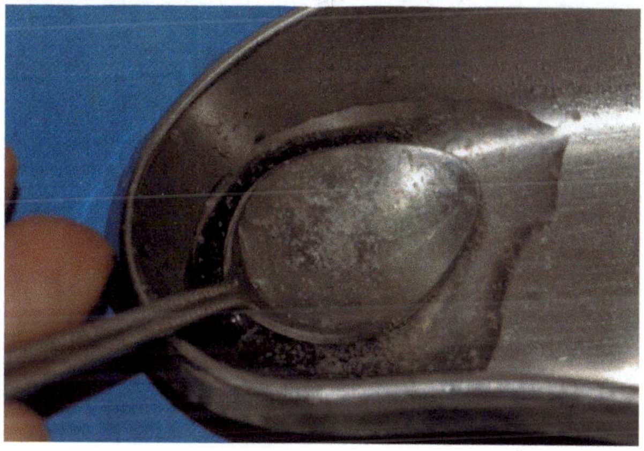

Fig. 15.5 Microskin grafts floated in normal saline in a kidney tray after preparing with the help of scissor

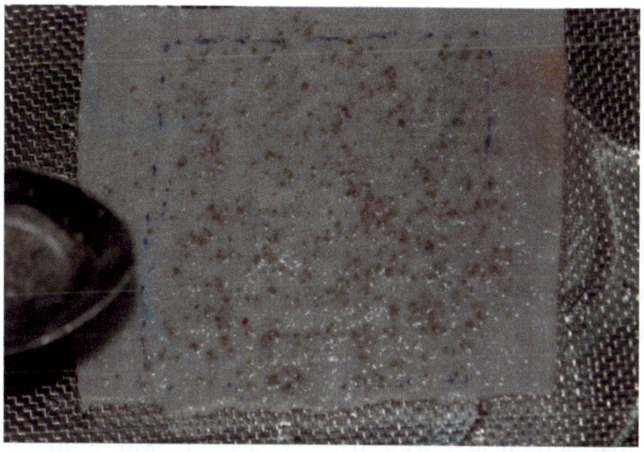

Fig. 15.6 Spreading of the MSGs on large square muslin sheet by a spoon

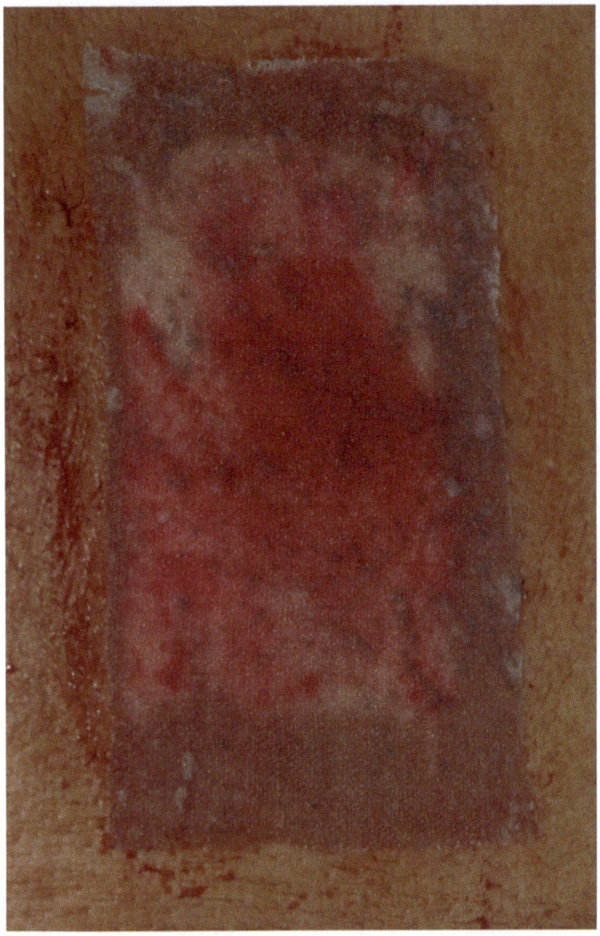

Fig. 15.7 Muslin sheet carrying the MSGs is applied on the dermabraded vitiliginous area on the back. The distributed MSGs can be seen through the muslin sheet

15.3 Microskin Grafting by Spraying Method in Extensive Vitiligo Management

Ultra thin or thin autologous skin from vitiligo patients was harvested and cut into pieces of 0.2–0.5 mm in size and suspended in normal saline. The suspension was put into a bottle with an outlet and a pumping device. The microskin suspended in the saline was sprayed to the abraded vitiliginous area and the microskin distribution was detected by digital image analysis technique. The area ratio of donor to recipient was 1:5–1:15 with spraying method. The advantages of this method are, well-distributed microskin, simpler handling, saving of donor skin, shortening of operating time and less time needed for wound healing and uniform pigmentation.

The technique has been successfully applied in all suitable patients with stable vitiligo and seems to be a simple and better alternative to tissue culture, for grafting extensive vitiliginous areas.

The aesthetic results were found to be better in the areas where microskin grafting was carried out, as compared to thin and ultra thin split thickness skin graft (STSG-T, STSG-UT). Also, large segments of micrografts are not compromised if a small area of MSG detached, and pigmentation is faster and more uniform. Microskin grafting can cover more area than sheet skin grafting, and subsequent PUVA treatment can enlarge the area of pigmentation with coalescence of adjacent grafts.

15.3.1 Variations in Spraying Method

- Spray MSGs on muslin sheet and then turn over it on abraded vitiliginous area
- Directly spray MSGs on the wound with the spraying device

15.3.1.1 Spray MSGs on Muslin Sheet and then Turn Over it on Abraded Vitiliginous Area (Figs. 15.8–15.10)

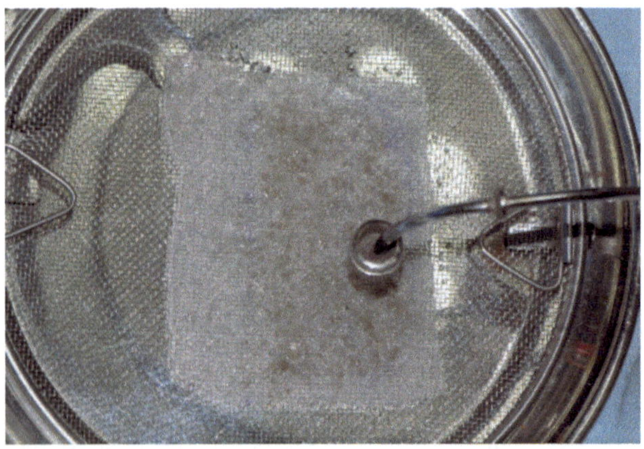

Fig. 15.8 MSGs sprayed on the muslin sheet by a spraying device

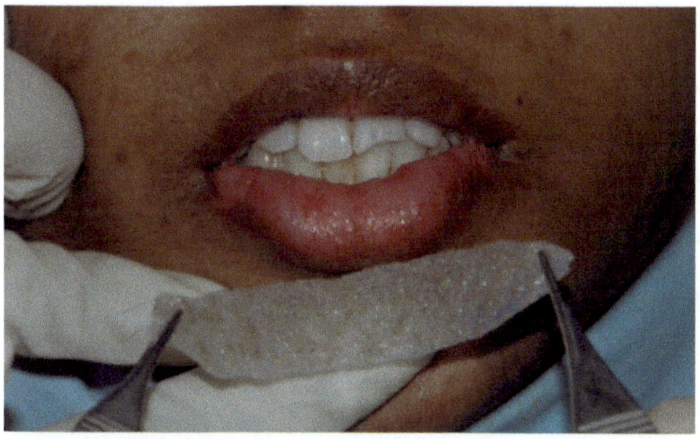

Fig. 15.9 Muslin sheet carrying the MSGs is cut according to the requirement and is being applied as shown on the lip

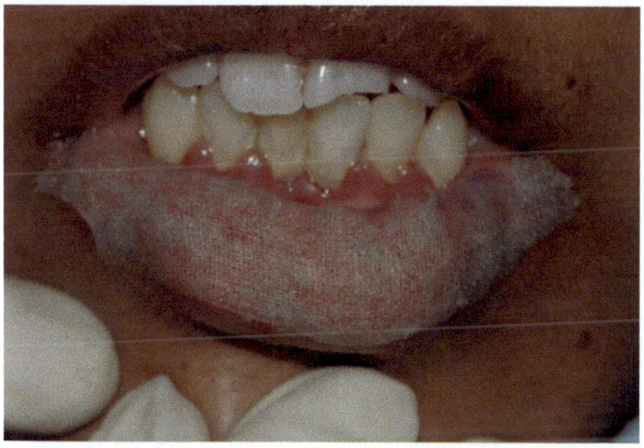

Fig. 15.10 Transplanted MSGs on the lower lip

15.3.1.2 Directly Spray on the Wound with the Pumping Device (Figs. 15.11–15.17)

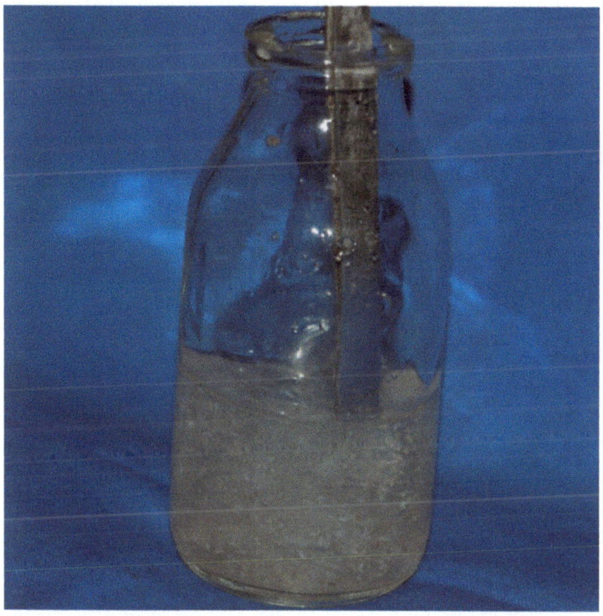

Fig. 15.11 The MSGs are stirred in small normal saline bottle

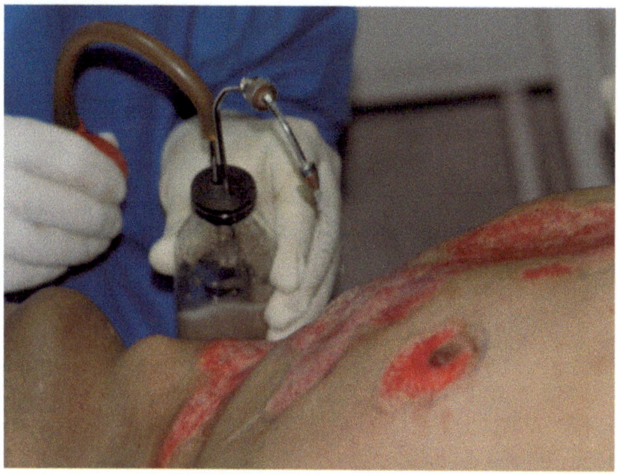

Fig. 15.12 Large dermabraded vitiliginous area on the chest is being sprayed directly by the MSGs with the help of a spraying device

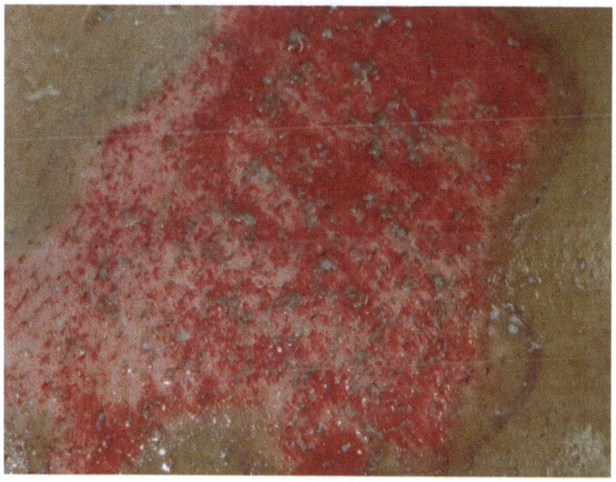

Fig. 15.13 Widely distributed MSGs on the chest by spraying device with good donor to recipient area expansion (1:15)

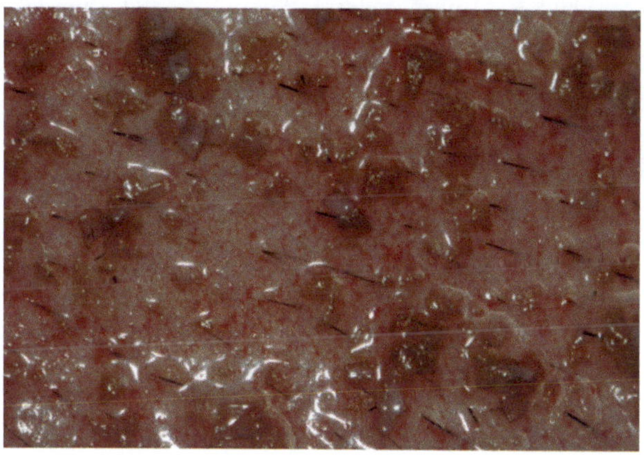

Fig. 15.14 Close up view of the distributed MSGs on dermabraded area

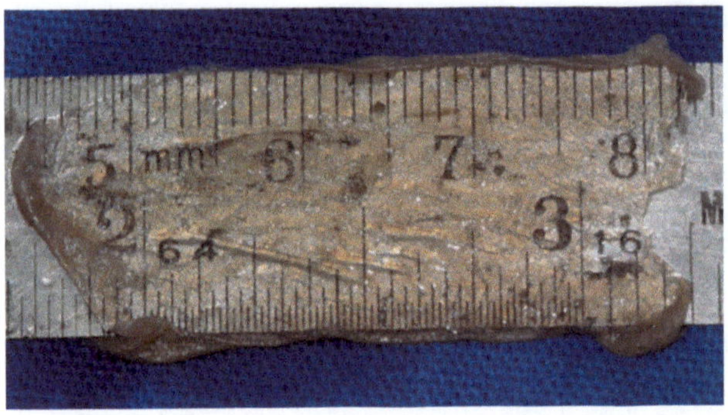

Fig. 15.15 Ultra thin split thickness skin graft (STSG-UT) is best for making MSGs and at the same time nearly avoids the donor area deformity

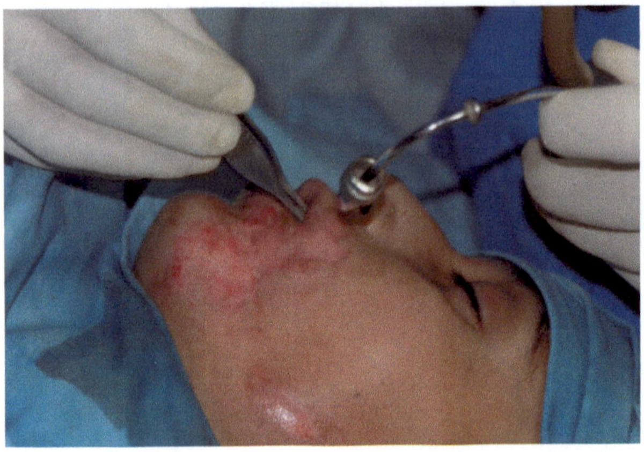

Fig. 15.16 MSGs are being sprayed on dermabraded vitiliginous area on the face

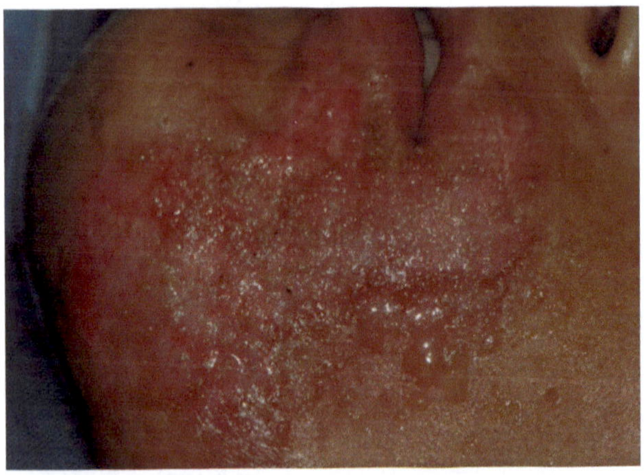

Fig. 15.17 Close up view of sprayed MSGs on the face

15.3.1.3 Comparison: Floatation vs. Spraying (Figs. 15.18–15.21)

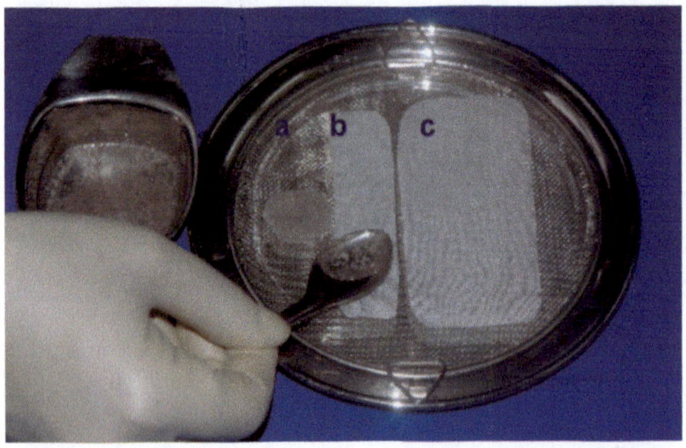

Fig. 15.18 Microskin grafts being dispersed on muslin cut sheets by a spoon (**a, b**). The larger muslin sheet will be sprayed by the MSGs by using spraying device for comparison(**c**)

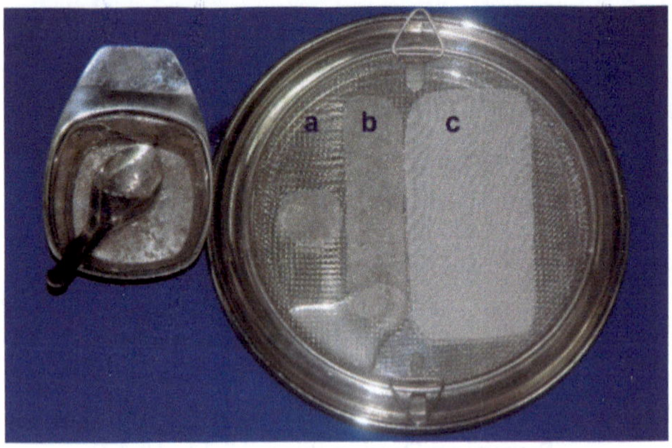

Fig. 15.19 Distribution of the MSGs on the first two smaller muslin cut sheets by a spoon (**a, b**). The larger muslin sheet will be sprayed by the MSGs by using spraying device for comparison (**c**)

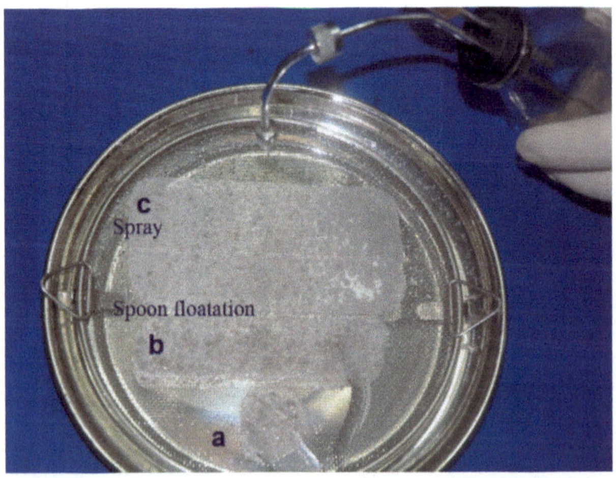

Fig. 15.20 Distribution of the MSGs on the first two smaller muslin cut sheets by a spoon (**a**, **b**). Microskin graft is being sprayed by spray device on large muslin sheet (**c**)

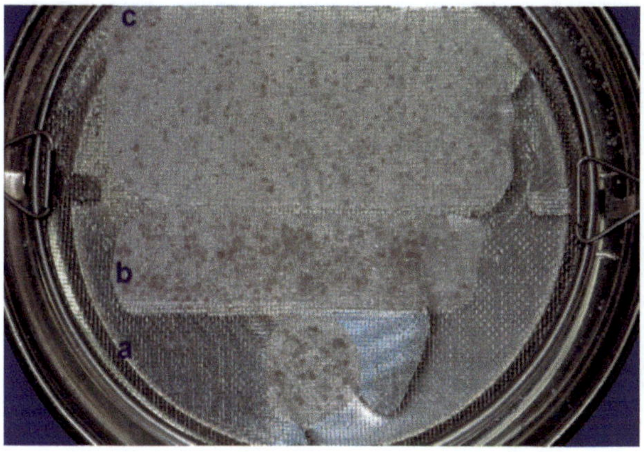

Fig. 15.21 Spoon distribution leads to conglomeration of the MSGs on the muslin sheet (**a, b**), while wide, nearly uniform distribution is achieved by spraying (**c**)

15.3.1.4 Turn Over (Reversing) the MSGs to Change Their Orientation

Epithelial side up vs. epithelial side down (Figs. 15.22–15.25).

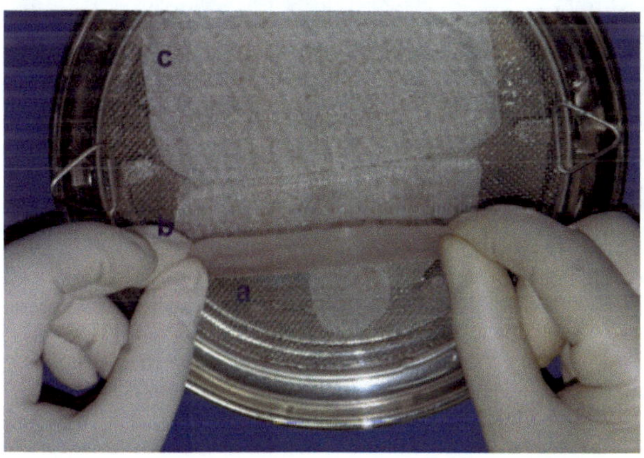

Fig. 15.22 In order to reverse the orientation of the MSGs, vaselined tulle gras is being laid down on the MSGs (**b**) already distributed on the muslin strip. On magnification if one notices the MSGs with more epithelial side up, then these can be reversed on vaselined muslin sheet, so that maximum graft with dermal sides come in contact with the vitiliginous dermabraded raw area to increase the survival of grafts. Shows distribution of MSGs on muslin sheet by spray device and spoon respectively (**c, a**)

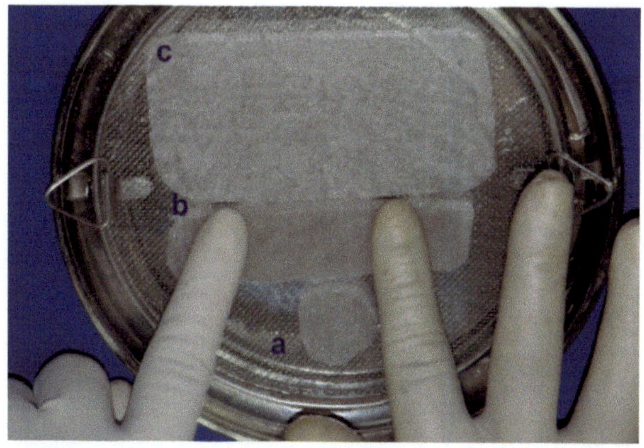

Fig. 15.23 Vaselined tulle gras being gently ironed with fingers (**b**). Shows distribution of MSGs on muslin sheet by spray device and spoon respectively (**c, a**)

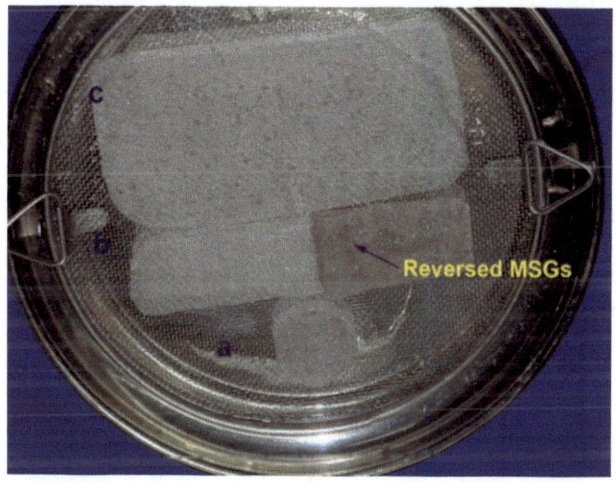

Fig. 15.24 MSGs are being transferred on vaselined muslin tulle gras (**b**). Shows distribution of MSGs on muslin sheet by spray device and spoon respectively (**c, a**)

Fig. 15.25 Close up view of reversed MSGs on vaselined tulle gras

15.3.1.5 **Points to be Noted** (Figs. 15.26–15.29)

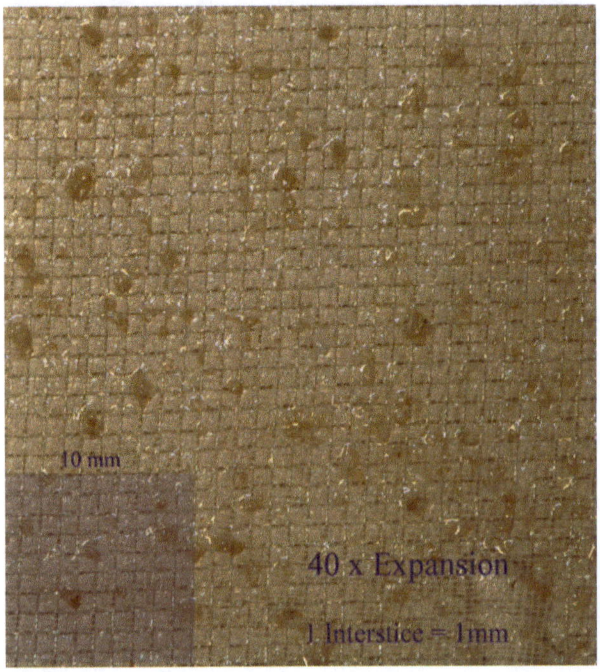

Fig. 15.26 Close up view of distributed MSGs on muslin sheet by spraying method (donor to recipient ratio 1:40). Expansion more than 1:15 may take a long time for complete repigmentation or may leave behind the skip vitiliginous areas. Quick and early repigmentation achieved with 1:5–1:15 donor to recipient area ratio in 6 months time

Fig. 15.27 Excessive spraying of MSGs at a point should be avoided. In this overcrowded MSGs, most of the grafts are facing with epithelial side up. These MSGs must be reversed on tulle gras before application to keep the dermal side of most of the MSGs in contact with the Vitiliginous raw area and thus increase the maximum chances of graft survival

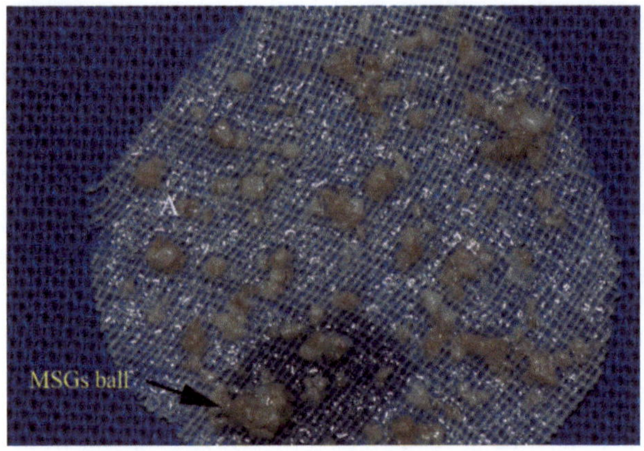

Fig. 15.28 Close up view of dispersed MSGs by a spoon on a small round piece of muslin. If the autografts are thicker, the minced skin tends to form small balls with the epithelial side outwards and thus, cannot survive on the wound

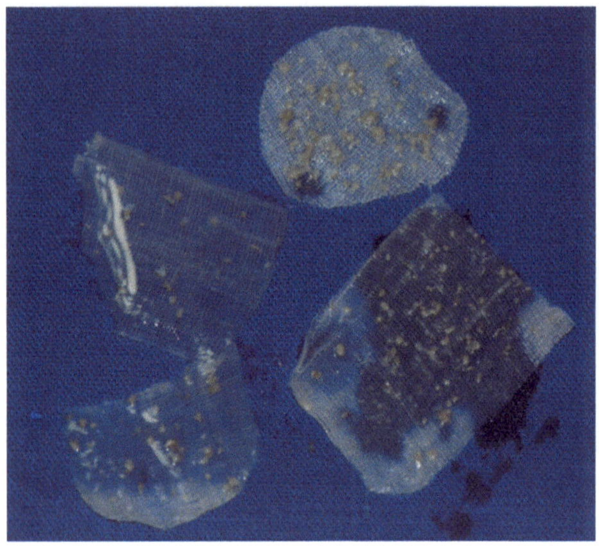

Fig. 15.29 Left over pieces of muslin, carrying MSGs, utilized for covering small isolated vitiliginous lesions for repigmentation

Part III

Step-by-Step Microskin Grafting Techniques

Microskin Grafting by Direct Spread Method 16

(Donor to recipient area expansion ratio 1:1)

With direct spread method, you need approximately 1:1 donor to recipient area ratio to repigment the vitiliginous area. It is the big drawback of this method. Repigmentation is very fast with good color match and uniformity. There is no failure in stable vitiligo and if it occurs, is the fault of proper execution of the technique, rather than the fault of the technique itself. Depigmentation occurs after the "take" of grafts only in active disease or the disease becomes active during treatment.

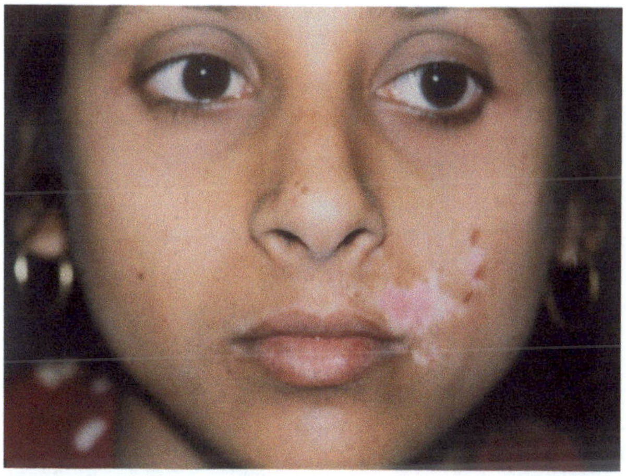

Fig. 16.1.1 Stable segmental vitiligo on the left side of cheek (my first case of Microskin grafting operated in 1995)

16.1 Case 1 (Segmental Vitiligo-Cheek)

I did my first case of segmental vitiligo left cheek in 1995. This STSG was taken from the gluteal region and cut into micro skin grafts with the help of scissors. Most of the skin particles were around 1 mm and the donor area used was a little more than the recipient area. Following dermabrasion with diamond fraise, the vitiliginous area was covered by thick layer microskin grafts. Microskin grafts took well . Most of the microskin grafts with epithelial side down were dried out and rejected. The microskin grafts that took well were so closely packed that nearly 70% of the vitiliginous area got pigmented in 30 days time.

In this patient, a little larger size of MSGs were used, leading to mild cobblestoning which disappeared after some time. This event taught me to make fine MSGs much smaller than 1 mm using thin or ultra thin split thickness skin graft (Figs. 16.1.1 and 16.1.2).

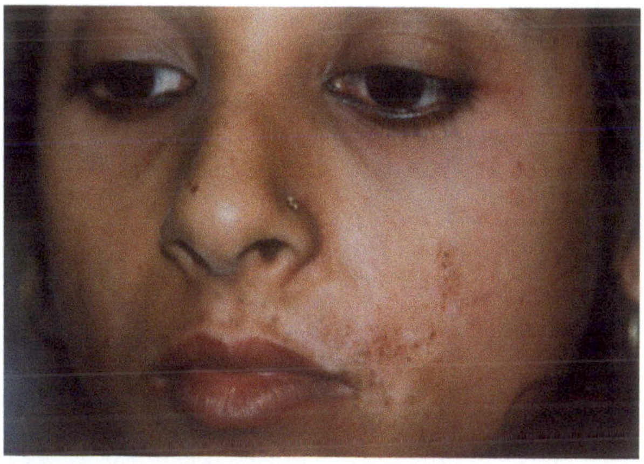

Fig. 16.1.2 Amount of repigmentation achieved after 1 month

D. K. Gupta, *Microskin Grafting for Vitiligo*,
DOI: 10.1007/978-1-84882-605-2_16, © Springer Science + Business Media B.V. 2009

16.2 Case 2 (Segmental Vitiligo-Left Upper Eyelid)

In this case of segmental vitiligo the left upper eyelid was managed by microskin grafting. Frontal nerve block was used to anesthetize the upper eyelid and local anesthetic infiltration (0.4% lidocaine) was done to anesthetize anterior axillary fold which was used as the donor area (Figs. 16.2.1–16.2.5).

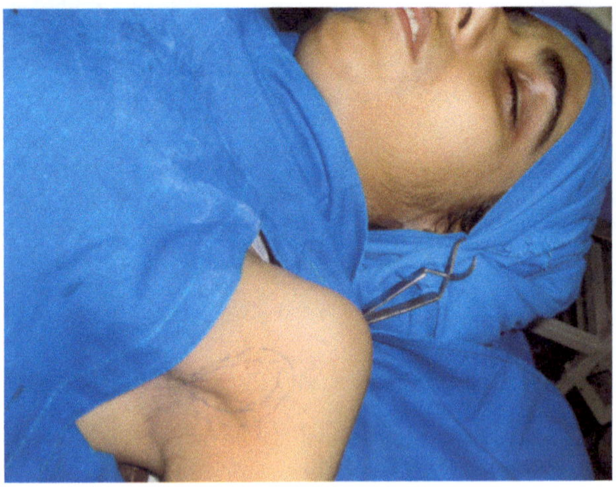

Fig. 16.2.1 Stable segmental vitiligo present on the left upper eyelid. Donor area marked on the left anterior axillary fold

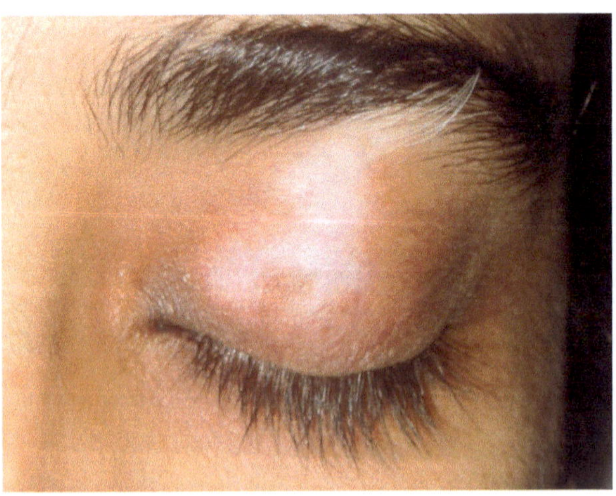

Fig. 16.2.2 Close up pre operative view of the upper left eyelid

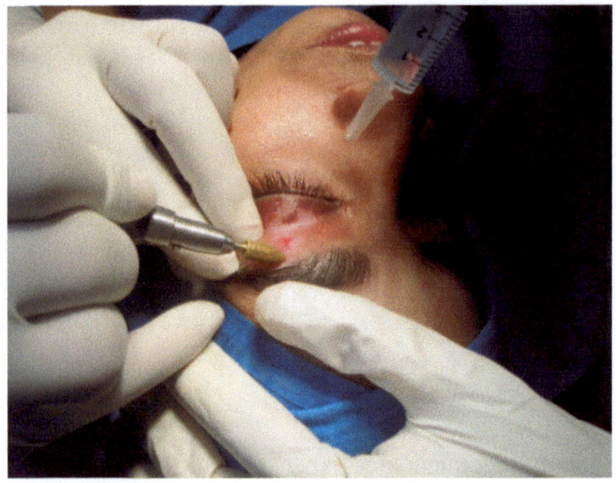

Fig. 16.2.3 Vitiliginous area superficially dermabraded with diamond fraise. The eyelid and the eyebrow kept stretched and continuously wetted with normal saline to avoid any thermal damage through friction

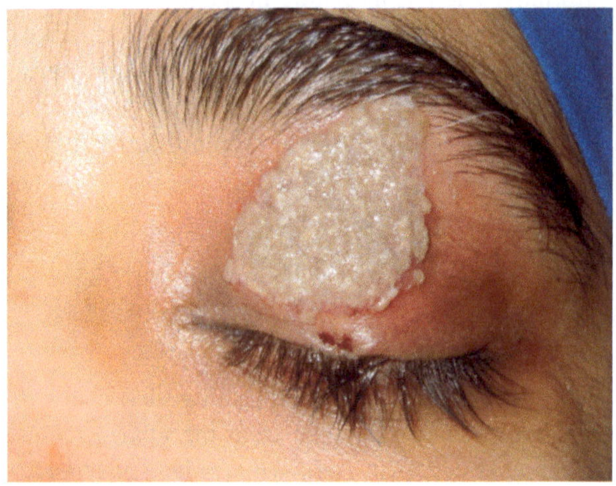

Fig. 16.2.4 Ultra thin microskin graft spread over abraded upper eyelid. Temporary central tarsorraphy for 5 days

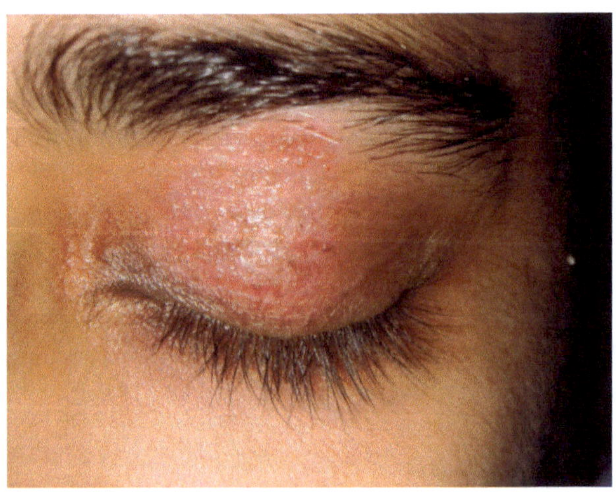

Fig. 16.2.5 Amount of repigmentation after 21 days of microskin grafting

16.3 Case 3 (Vitiligo Vulgaris-Right Foot) (Figs. 16.3.1–16.3.2)

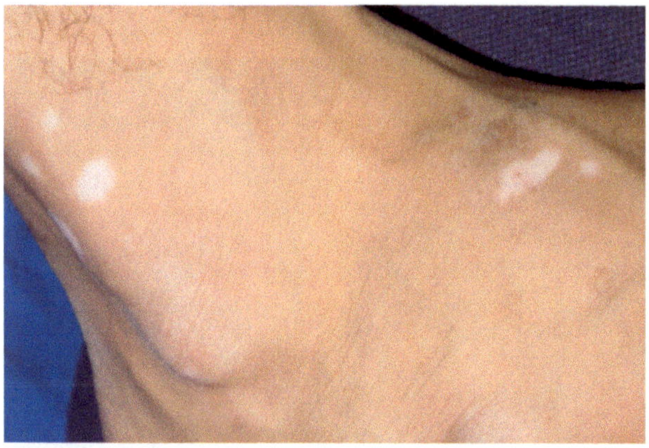

Fig. 16.3.1 Stable vitiligo on foot

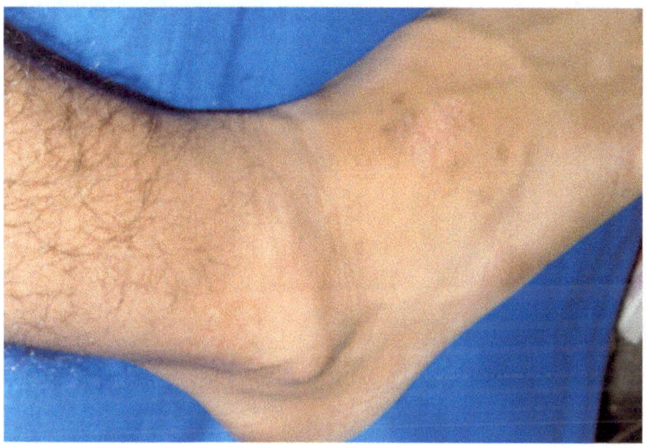

Fig. 16.3.2 Almost complete repigmentation after 42 days of MSGs

16.4 Case 4 (Palmer Vitiligo-Left Hand) (Figs. 16.4.1–16.4.4)

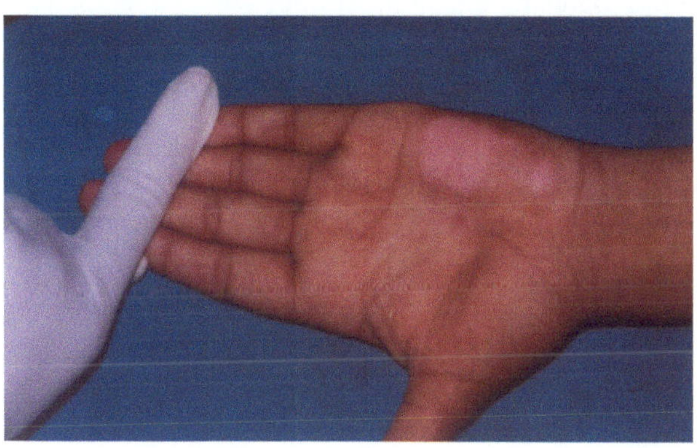

Fig. 16.4.1 Palmer vitiligo (left hand)

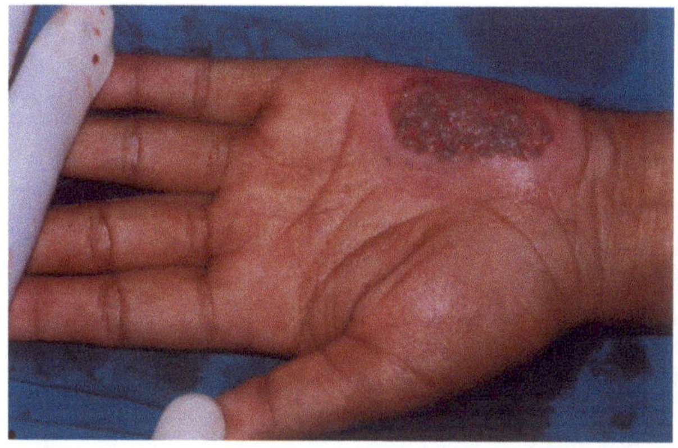

Fig. 16.4.2 After dermabrasion, microskin grafts were spread over the vitiliginous area of the palm

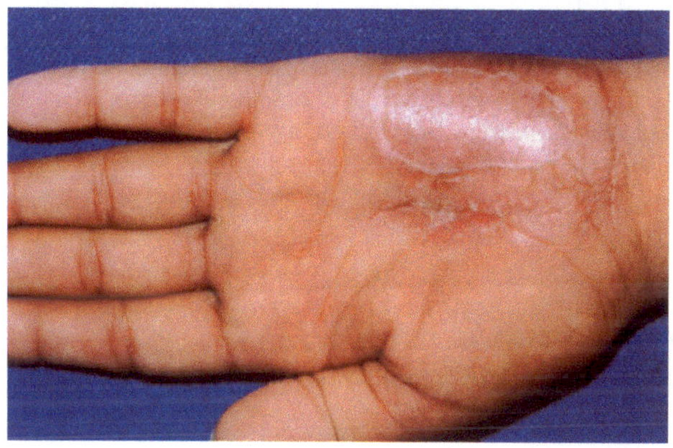

Fig. 16.4.3 On the 21st post operative day, wound got fully epithelized and the quantity of repigmentation is remarkable

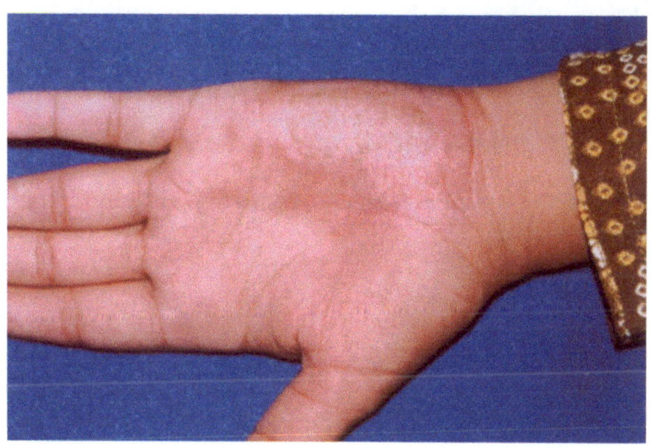

Fig. 16.4.4 Complete repigmentation achieved. Mild Cobblestoning noticed due to use of slightly bigger microskin grafts

16.5 Case 5 (Bindi Leukoderma-Contact Depigmentation from Adhesive) (Figs. 16.5.1–16.5.2)

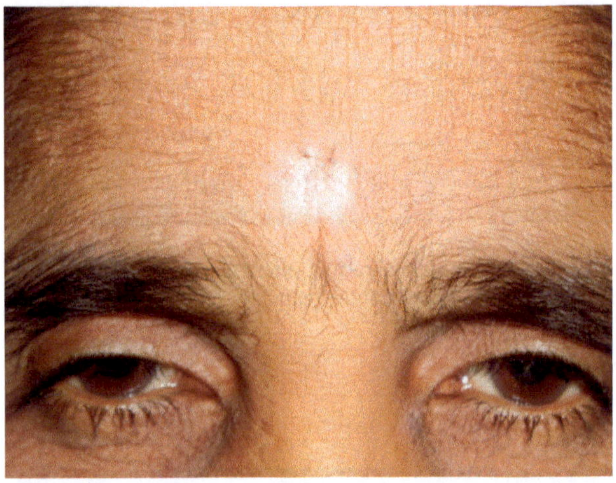

Fig. 16.5.1 Bindi (a circular beautification thing to be stuck on the forehead just above the root of nose) Leukoderma. Contact depigmentation from free paratertiary – butylphenol in bindi adhesive

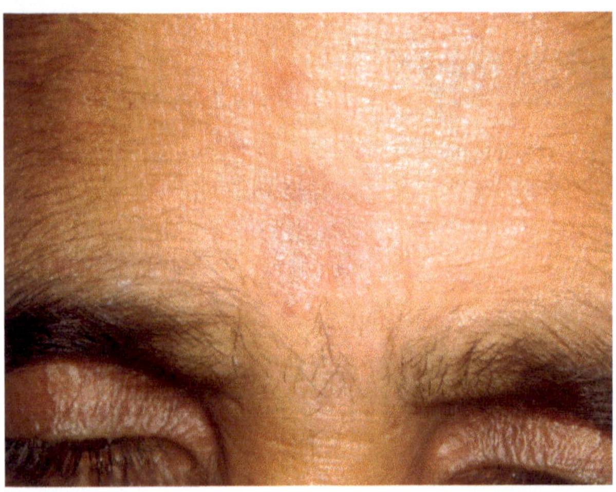

Fig. 16.5.2 On second month post operative: complete repigmentation

16.6 Case 6 (Vitiligo-Right Foot) (Figs. 16.6.1–16.6.5)

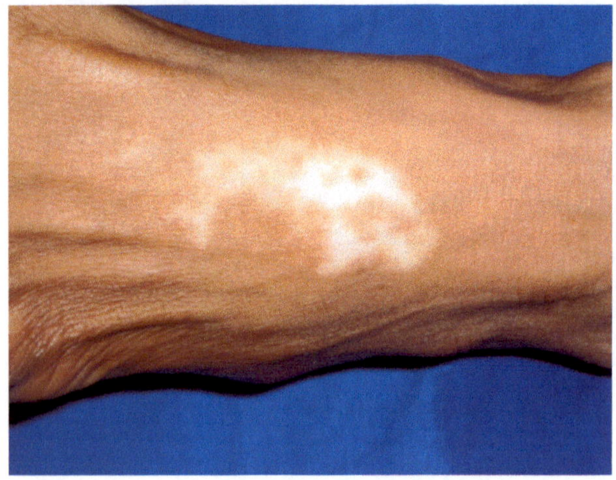

Fig. 16.6.1 Stable vitiligo on foot

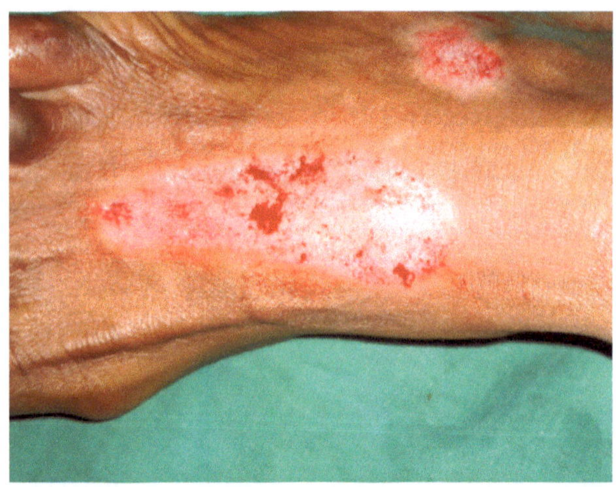

Fig. 16.6.2 Mixed superficial and accidental deep dermabrasion

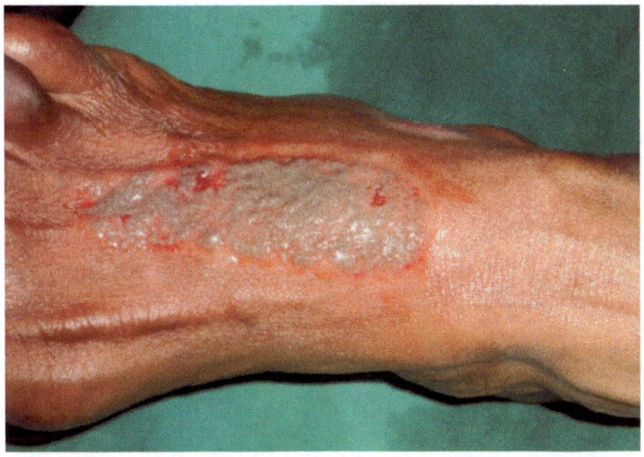

Fig. 16.6.3 Microskin grafting over abraded area

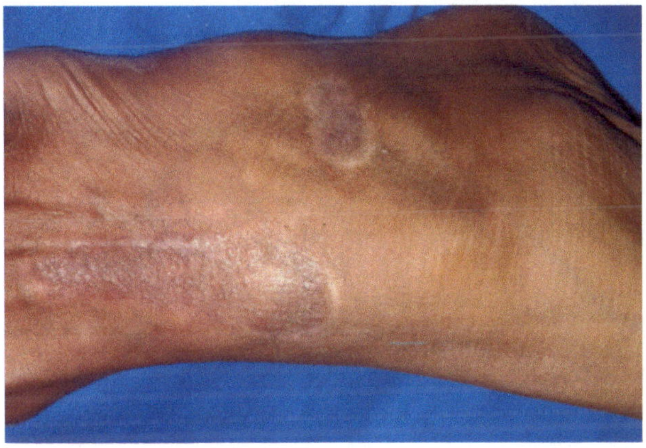

Fig. 16.6.4 On 27th post operative day

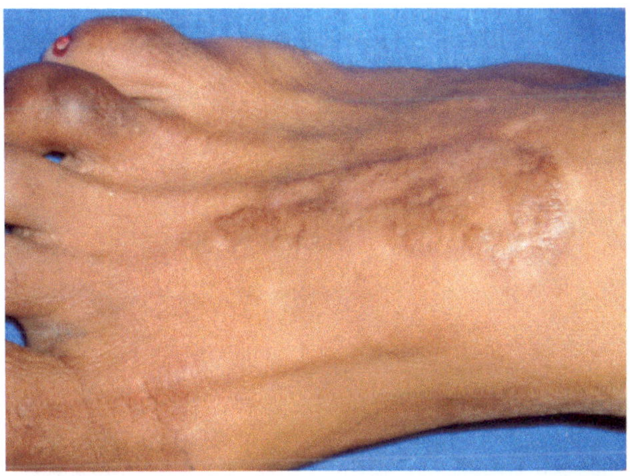

Fig. 16.6.5 On 56th post operative day: complete repigmentation and hypertrophic scar formation at places of accidental deep dermabrasion

16.7 Case 7 (Segmental Vitiligo-Right Side of Face) (Figs. 16.7.1 and 16.7.2)

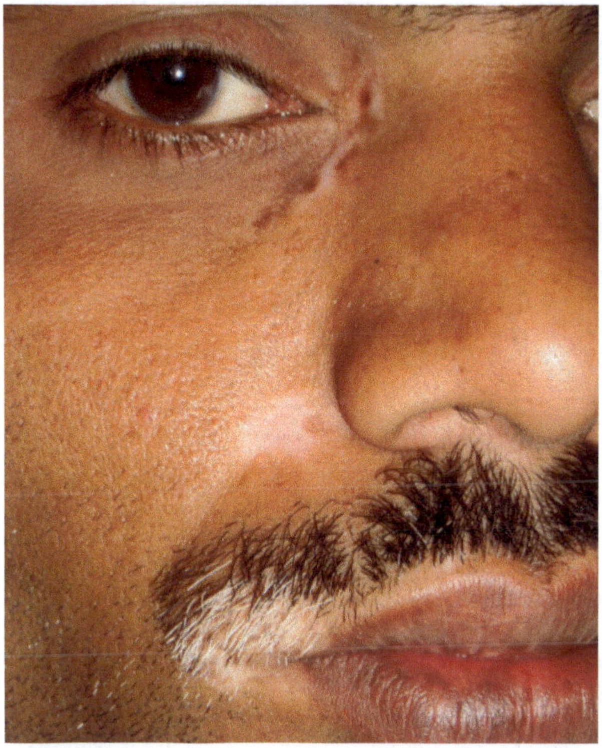

Fig. 16.7.1 Stable segmental vitiligo on right side of the face

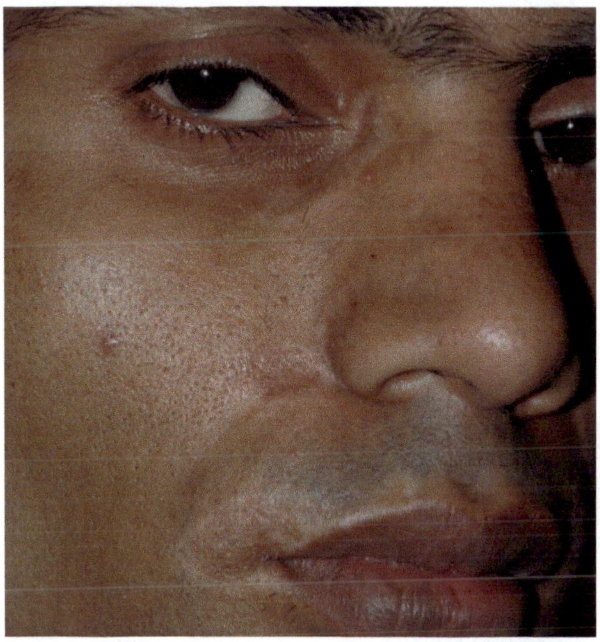

Fig. 16.7.2 Forty-five days post MSGs transplantation, almost complete repigmentation

16.8 Case 8 (Segmental Vitiligo-Forehead) (Figs. 16.8.1–16.8.3

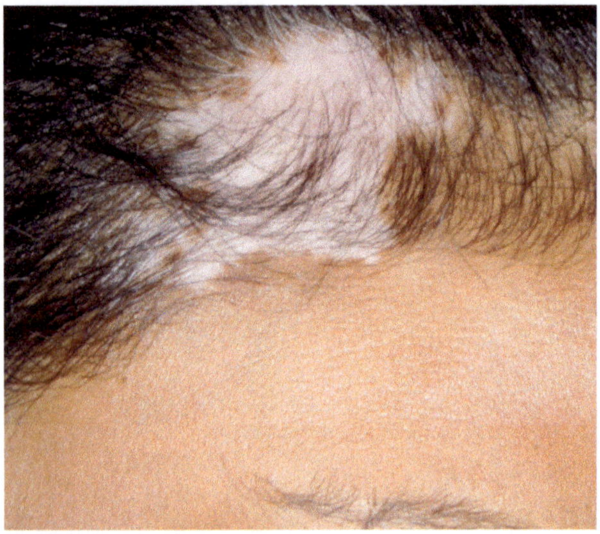

Fig. 16.8.1 Stable focal vitiligo on the right side of the forehead near hair line

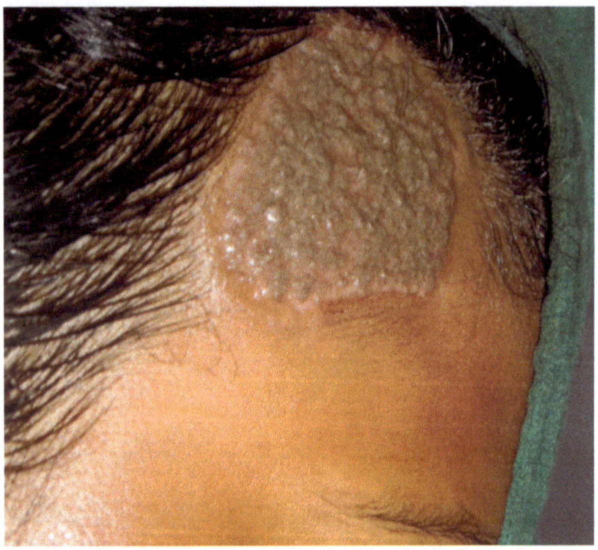

Fig. 16.8.2 Microskin grafting

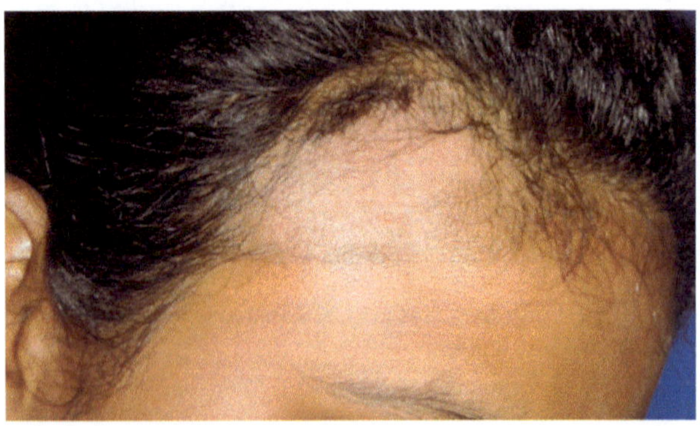

Fig. 16.8.3 Results at 37 days, almost complete repigmentation

16.9 Case 9 (Segmental Vitiligo-Left Cheek) (Figs. 16.9.1–16.9.3)

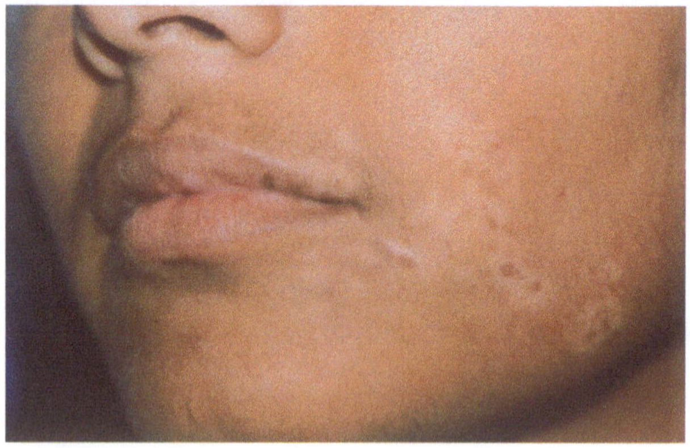

Fig. 16.9.1 The patient with residual patches of vitiligo following medical treatment on left side of the cheek

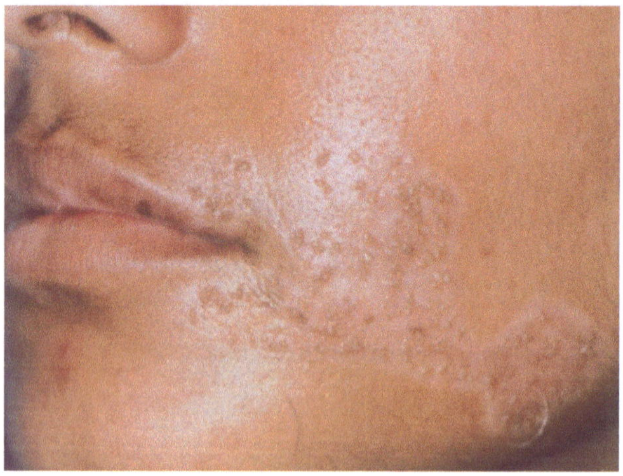

Fig. 16.9.2 Relatively larger and thicker size microskin grafts used. Mild cobblestoning noticed

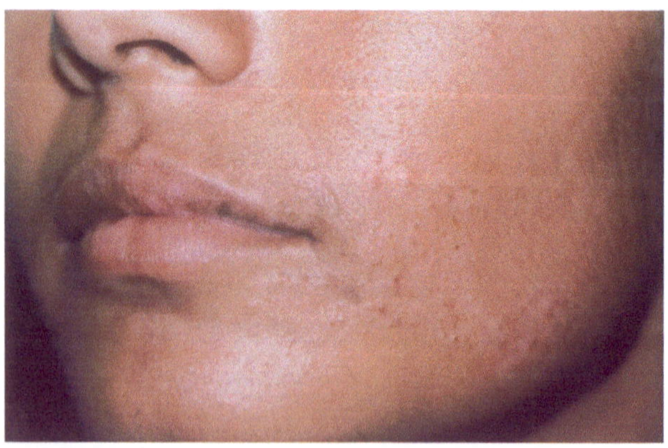

Fig. 16.9.3 Cobblestoning nearly disappeared and good colour match achieved at 3 months

16.10 Case 10 (Segmental Vitiligo-Left Eyebrow and Forehead) (Figs. 16.10.1–16.10.3)

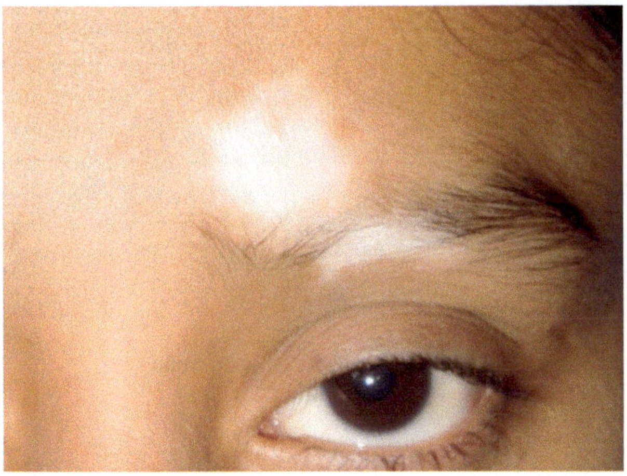

Fig. 16.10.1 Stable segmental vitiligo on left side of the eyebrow and the forehead

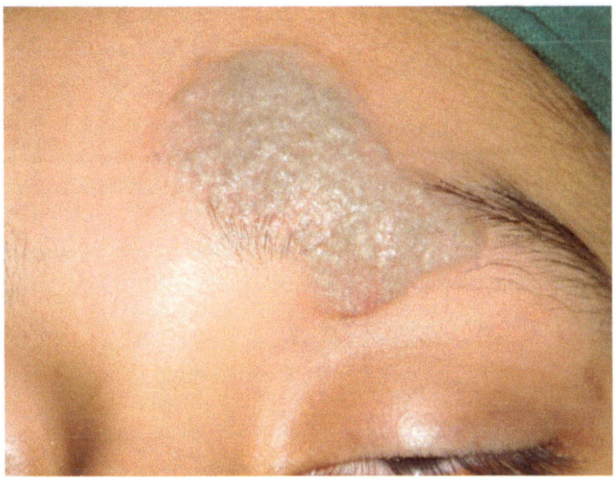

Fig. 16.10.2 Microskin grafting

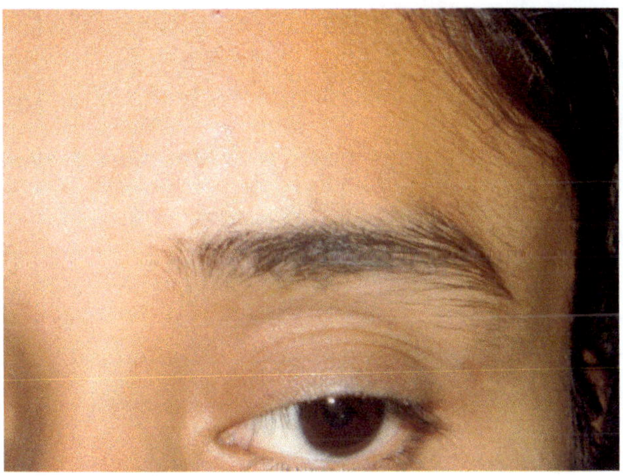

Fig. 16.10.3 Excellent repigmentation and color match after 4 months. Leukotrichia also recovered

16.11 Case 11 (Vitiligo-Fingers of Both Hands) (Figs. 16.11.1–16.11.4)

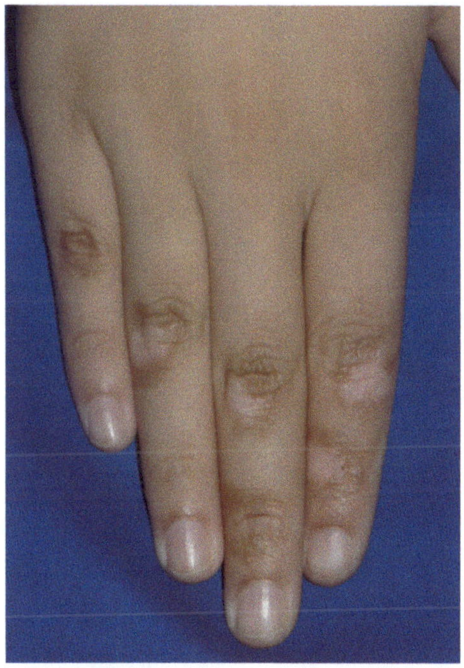

Fig. 16.11.1 Stable vitiligo on fingers of right hand

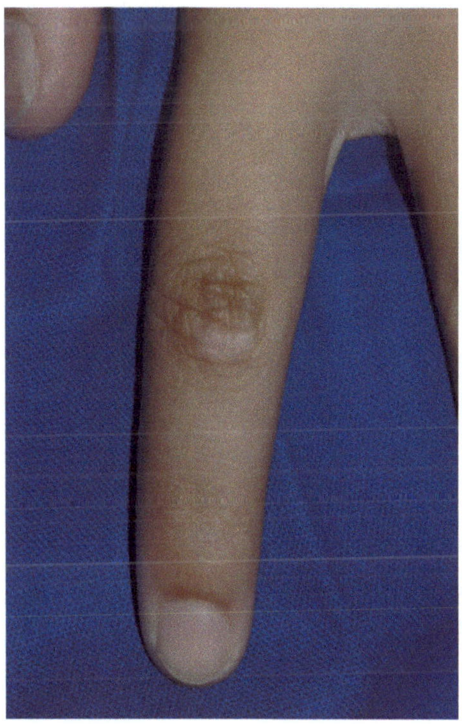

Fig.16.11.2 Stable vitiligo on left index fingers at proximal interphalangeal joint

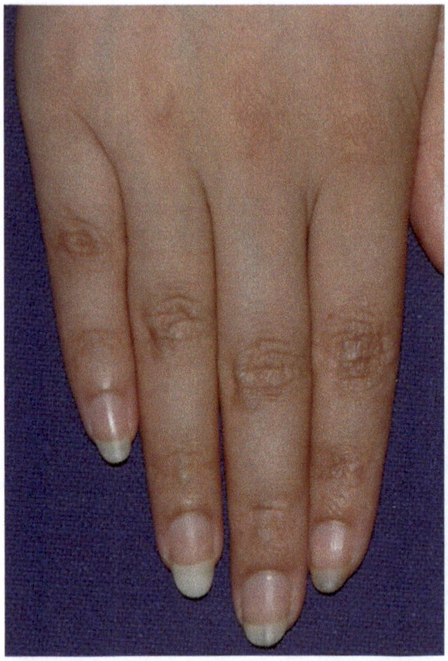

Fig. 16.11.3 Eleven months post microskin grafting, Complete repigmentation and excellent color match

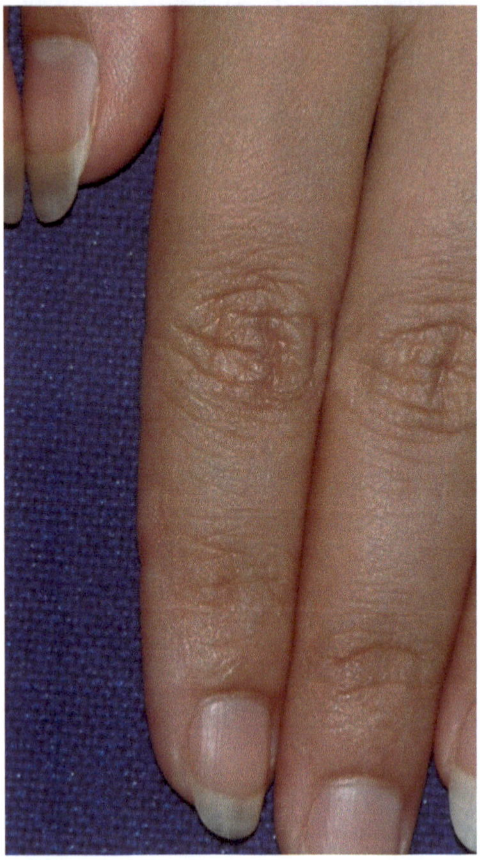

Fig. 16.11.4 Complete repigmentation and excellent color match

16.12 Case 12 (Vitiligo-Upper Eyelids) (Figs. 16.12.1–16.12.2)

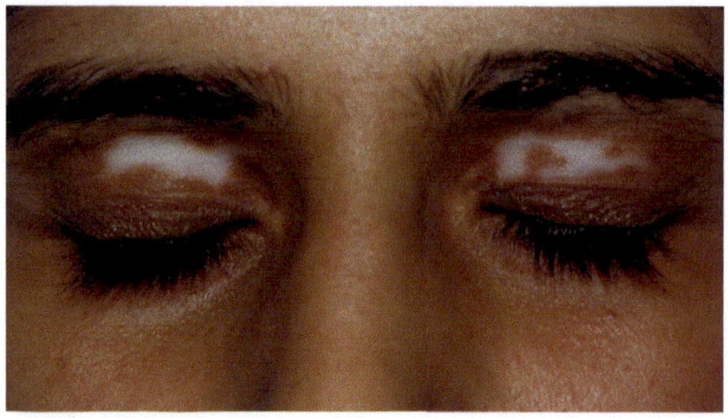

Fig. 16.12.1 Stable vitiligo on both upper eyelids

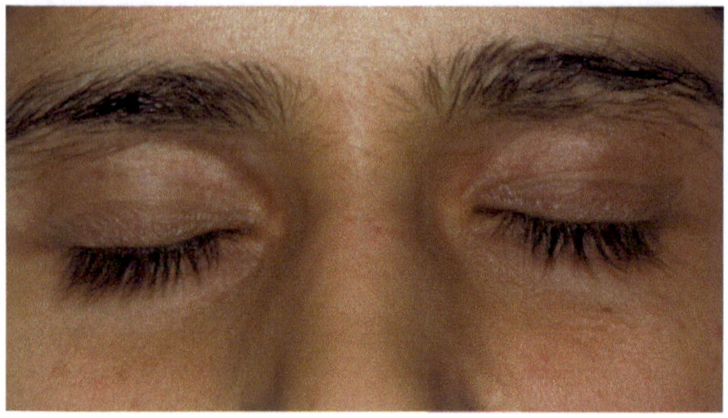

Fig. 16.12.2 At 45th post operative day, almost complete repigmentation

16.13 Case 13 (Naevus Depigmentosus) (Figs. 16.13.1–16.13.4)

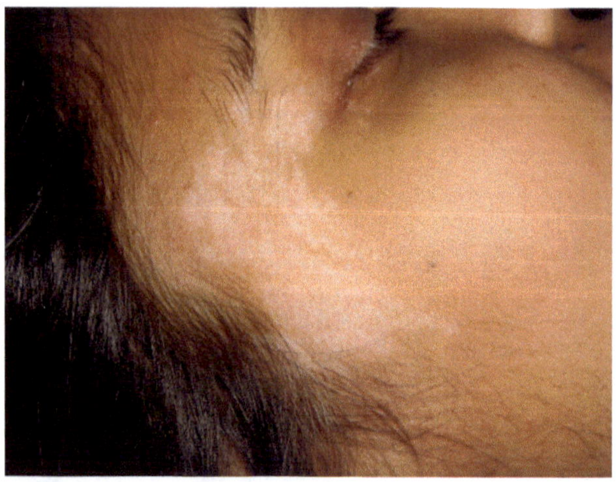

Fig. 16.13.1 Naevus depigmentosus

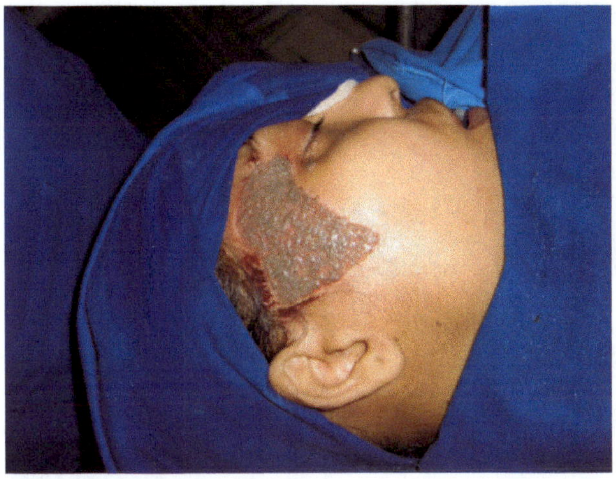

Fig. 16.13.2 Microskin grafting

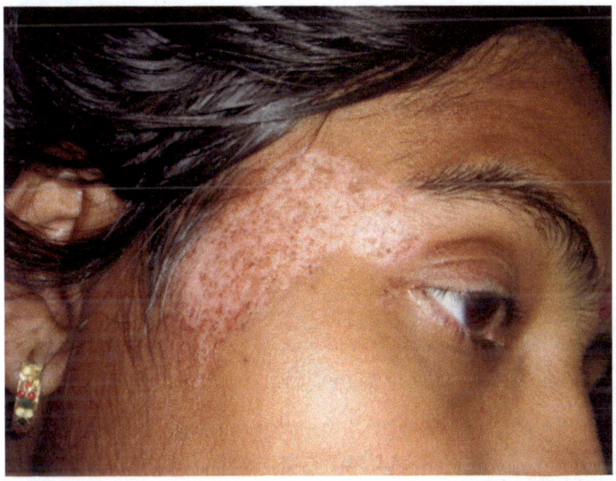

Fig. 16.13.3 Fifty days after operation: microskin grafts had been taken well but pigmentation did not spread

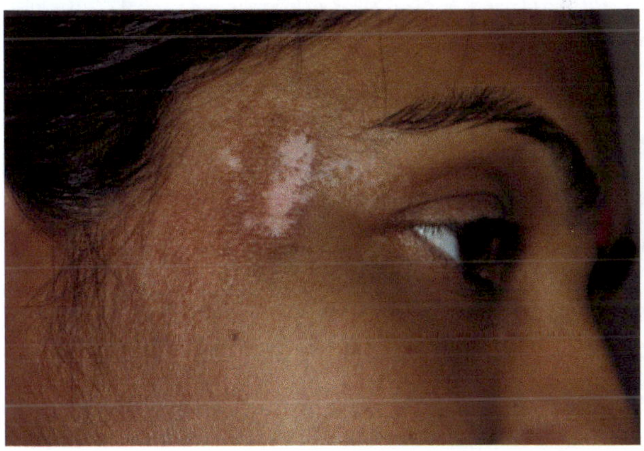

Fig. 16.13.4 At 22 months post operative: about 80% of the area pigmented. Naevus depigmentosus takes long time to get completely pigmented as in this case

16.14 Case 14 (Post Burn Dyschromia-Right Side of Face) (Figs. 16.14.1–16.14.6)

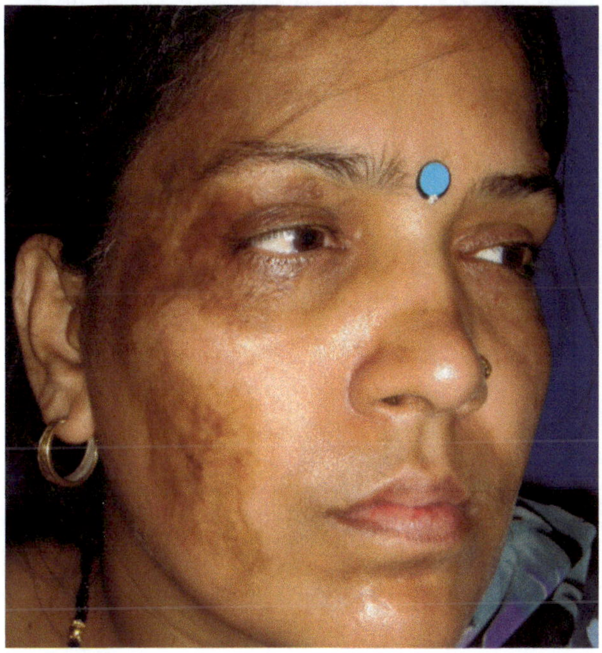

Fig. 16.14.1 Post burn hyperpigmented scar right side of the face

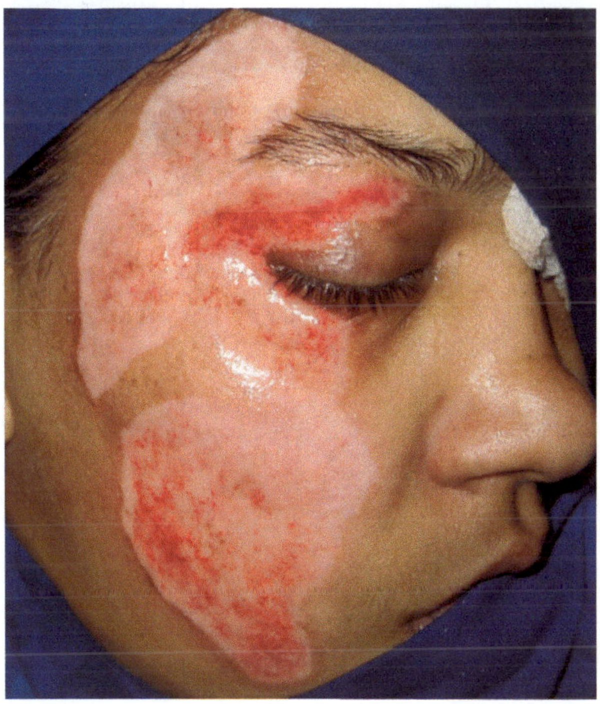

Fig. 16.14.2 Hyperpigmented area was superficially dermabraded with diamond fraise. Avoid catching in and pulling of the eyelashes and the eyebrow from moving fraise

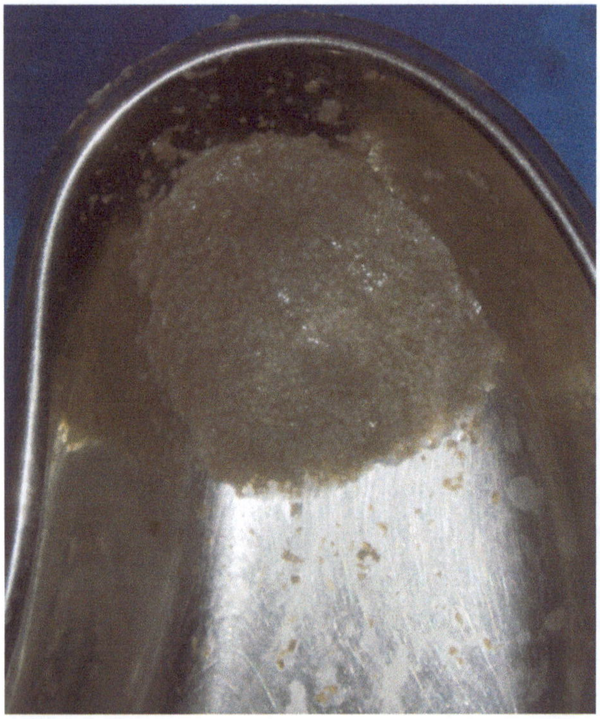

Fig. 16.14.3 Prepared microskin grafts

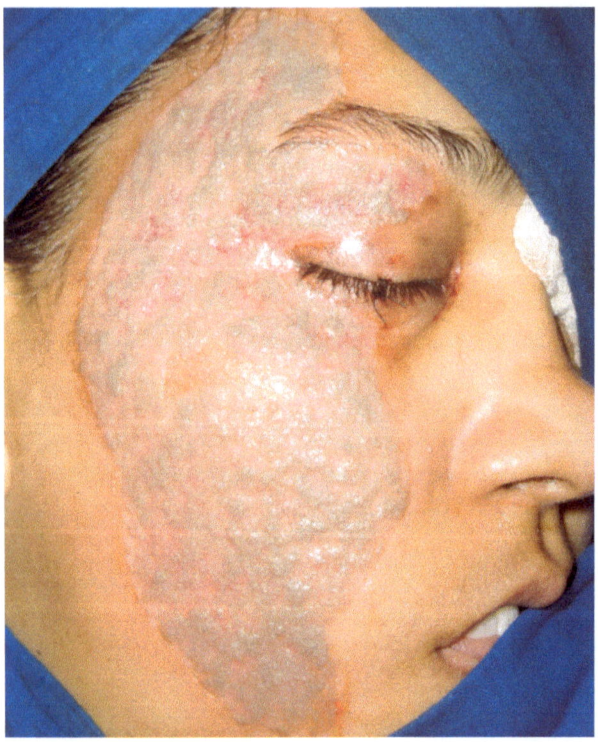

Fig. 16.14.4 Microskin graft spread on the previously abraded hyperpigmented area

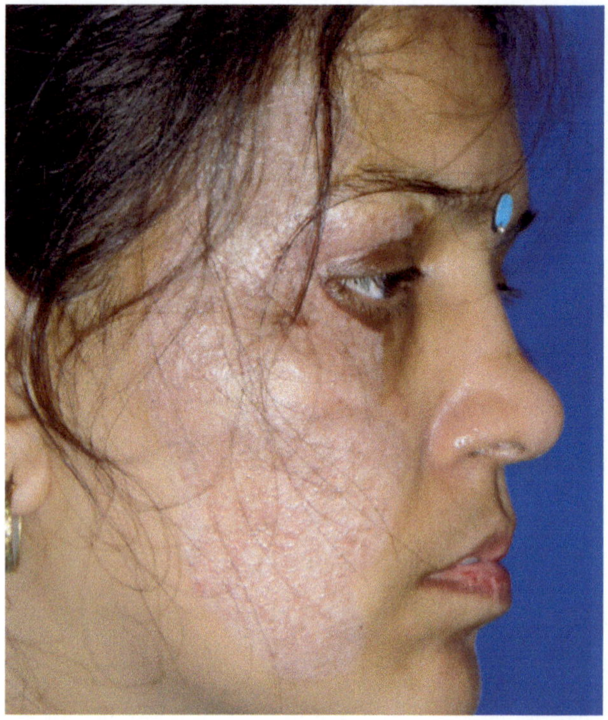

Fig. 16.14.5 Sixteenth post operative day: good repigmentation

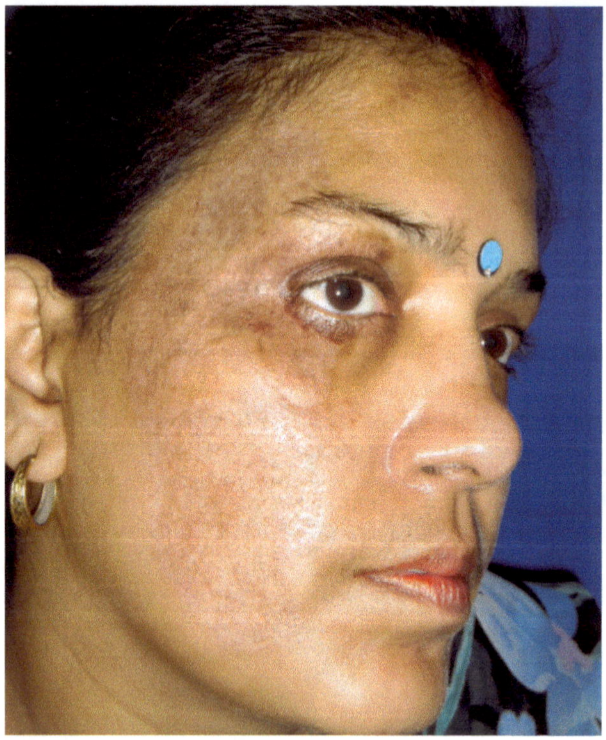

Fig. 16.14.6 Twenty-seventh post operative day: inclining towards fine color matching. Patient is advised to avoid sun exposure

Microskin Grafting by Floatation Method 17

(Donor to recipient area expansion ratio is about 1:3–1:10)

This method is applicable for a very small to a large vitiliginous area. Up to 1:10 donor to recipient area expansion can be achieved by floating the MSGs in normal saline and then spreading them on the muslin cloth sheet with the help of the spoon.

Pigmentary response is excellent with 1:3–1:5 expansion ratio. The vitiliginous area get pigmented in 3–4 months time and ultimately lead to good color match with the surrounding skin in a few months.

17.1 Case 1 (Post Burn Leukoderma: Cheek) (Figs. 17.1.1–17.1.3)

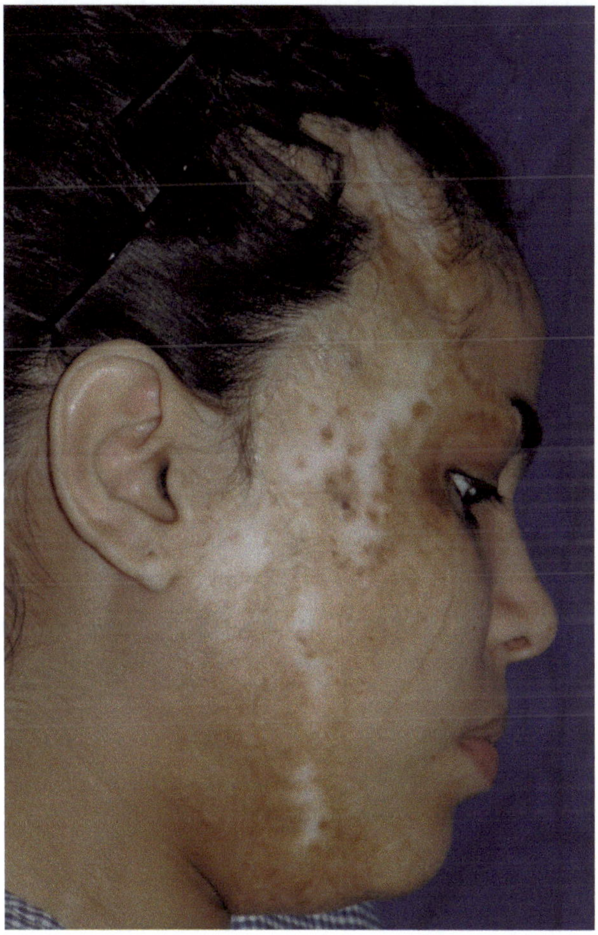

Fig. 17.1.1 Post burn depigmented and hyperpigmented scar on the right side of the face

D. K. Gupta, *Microskin Grafting for Vitiligo*,
DOI: 10.1007/978-1-84882-605-2_17, © Springer Science + Business Media B.V. 2009

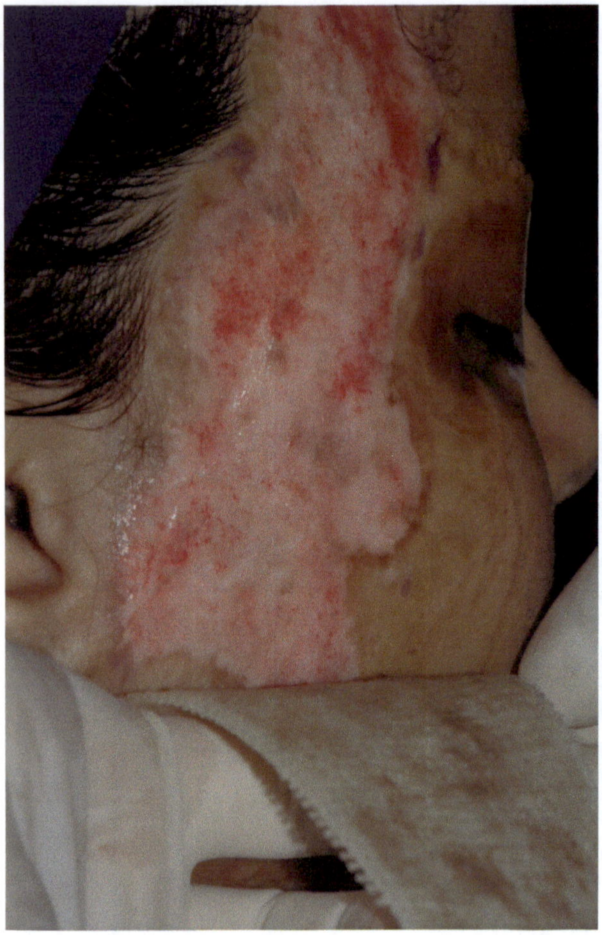

Fig. 17.1.2 Superficial dermabrasion done using diamond fraise. Dermabraded area of the cheek covered with tulle gras carrying microskin grafts (MSGs) on its deep surface. These MSGs first floated in normal saline, then dispersed on the muslin cloth by using a spoon and finally turned over the tulle gras

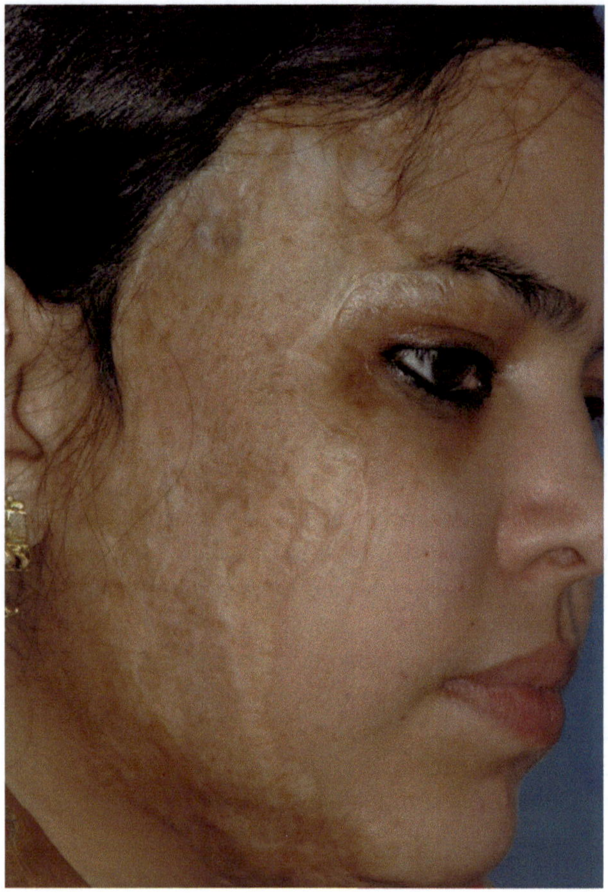

Fig. 17.1.3 Ninetieth post operative day–remarkable color match

17.2 Case 2 (Vitiligo Vulgaris) (Figs. 17.2.1–17.2.15)

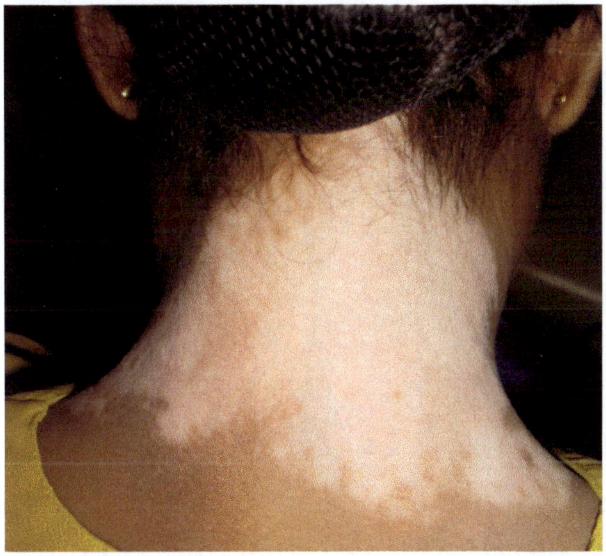

Figs. 17.2.1 A case of vitiligo vulgaris involving neck, eyelids, hands, elbows and feet. The vitiligo was managed elsewhere by 4 mm diameter punch grafts on neck, hand and feet. The picture shows depigmentation of punch grafts on the nape. She was planned for microskin grafting on eyelids, nape and sides of neck when the lesion again became stable and restarts pigmentation

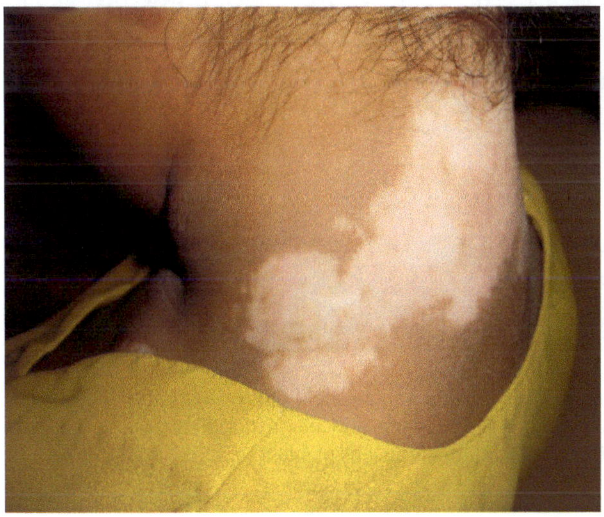

Figs. 17.2.2 The picture of same patient shows depigmentation of punch grafts on the nape and spreading of vitiliginous area

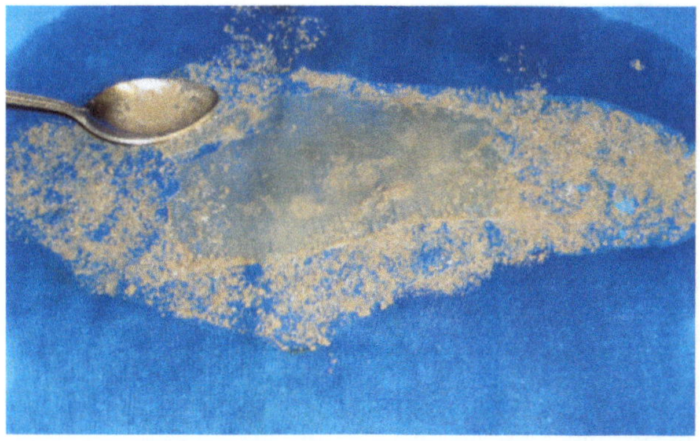

Fig. 17.2.3 Nape dermabraded by diamond fraise. Sterilized cotton cloth is used to take the imprint of the dermabraded area to make a template of raw area. In the center of the template, Ultra thin skin graft is spread out with epidermal side up. The rest of the area of template is covered by microskin grafts. The microskin grafts sprinkled with the help of tea spoon. The ultra thin graft and microskin grafts are turned over on dual layered vaseline impregnated tulle gras and applied over the dermabraded nape

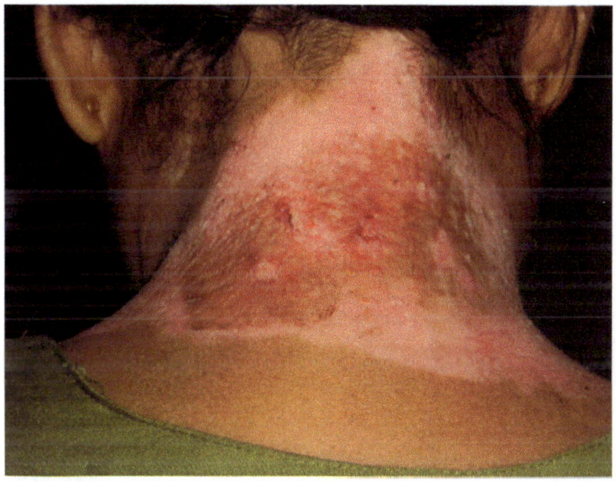

Fig. 17.2.4 Seventeenth post operative day: near total "take" of ultra thin and microskin grafts on nape

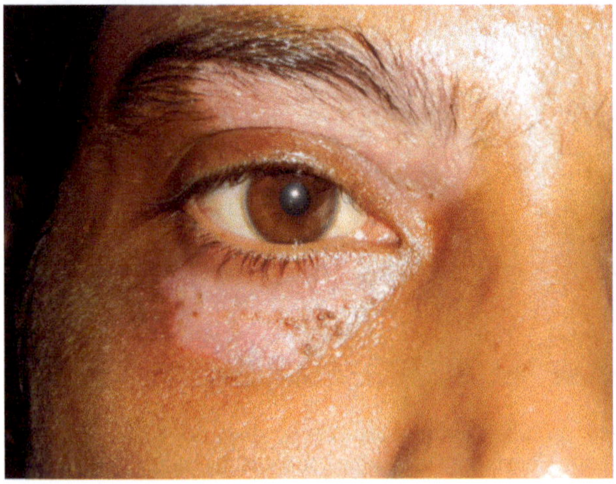

Figs. 17.2.5 The same patient on forty-fifth post operative day: photograph show rejection of the grafts and depigmentation of the eyelids. This indicates the activation of the disease process. She was kept on oral mini pulse (OMP) therapy by using 5 mg of betamethasone on two consecutive days in a week. Little puffiness on the face and weight gain noticed. This dose worked effectively in controlling the active disease process

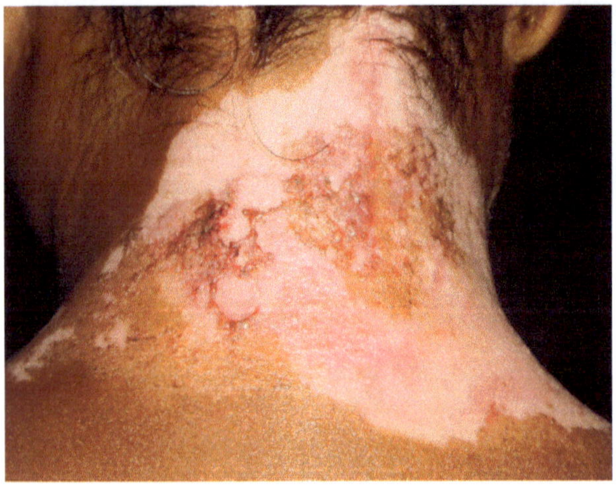

Figs. 17.2.6 Forty-fifth post operative day: photograph show rejection of the grafts and depigmentation of the nape

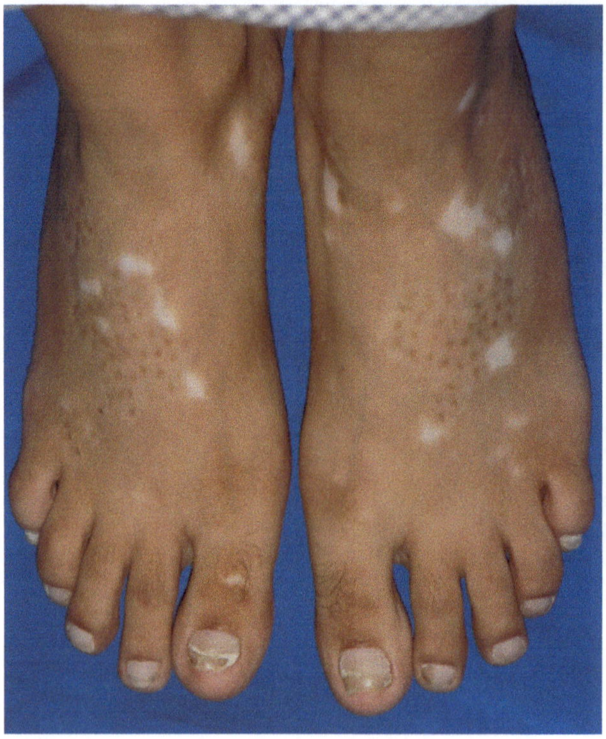

Figs. 17.2.7 In the same patient depigmentation arrested and disease again became stable. The residual vitiliginous areas on the feet, following previous 4 mm diameter punch graft. Residual vitiliginous lesions planned for microskin grafting

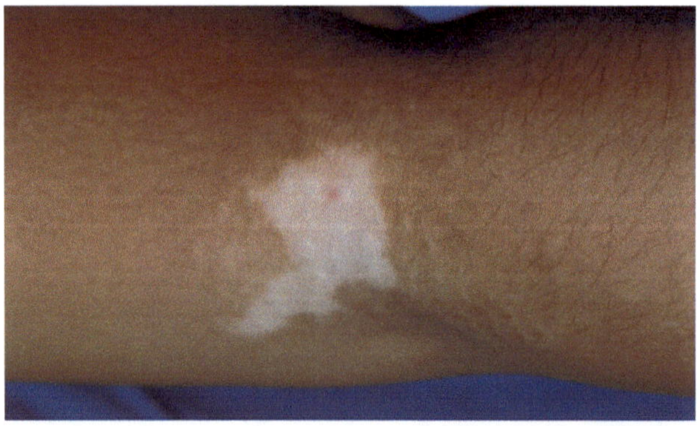

Figs. 17.2.8 In the same patient the residual vitiliginous areas on the elbow following previous 4 mm diameter punch graft. Residual vitiliginous lesions planned for microskin grafting

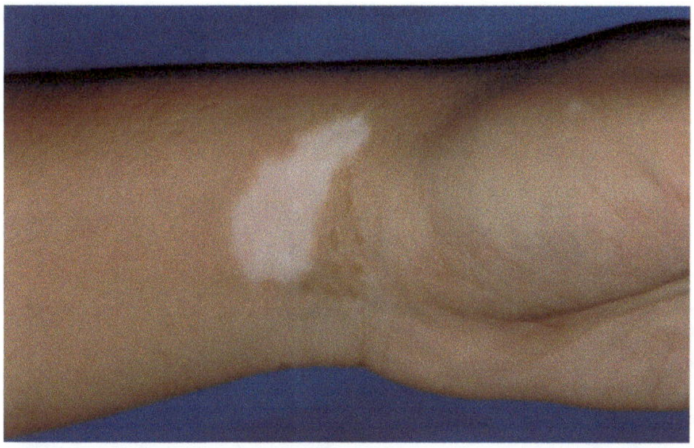

Figs. 17.2.9 In the same patient the residual vitiliginous areas on the wrist following previous 4 mm diameter punch graft. Residual vitiliginous lesions planned for microskin grafting

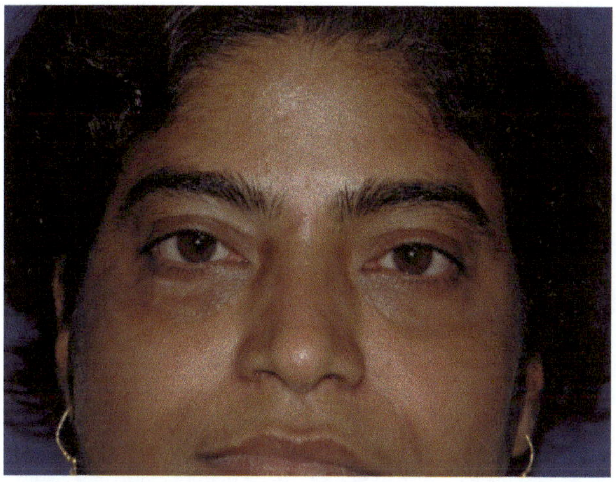

Fig. 17.2.10 Ninth post operative month – remarkable repigmentation of the right upper and lower eyelids after repeat microskin grafting on the eyelids

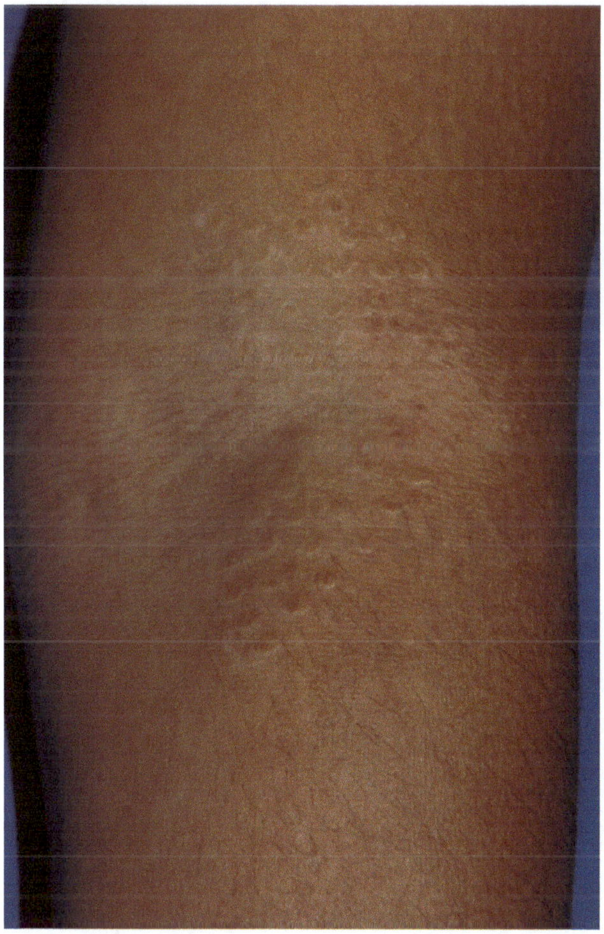

Figs. 17.2.11 Twenty-second month after microskin graft on residual lesion on the elbow. Normal pigmentation with excellent color match of the elbow. Cobblestoning of previous punch grafts also minimized to a great extent by dermabrasion and microskin grafting

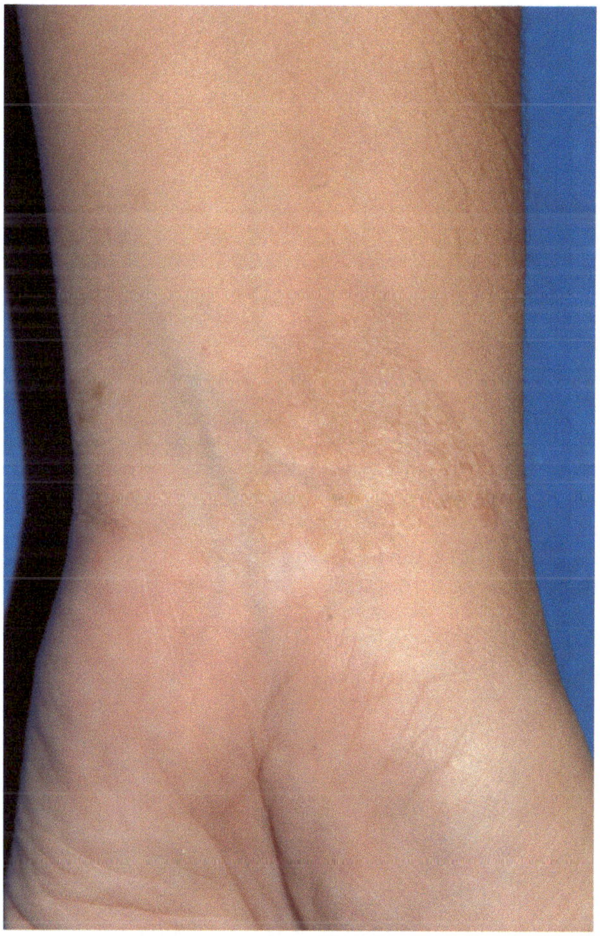

Figs. 17.2.12 Twenty-second month after microskin graft on residual lesion on the wrist. Normal pigmentation with excellent color match. Cobblestoning of previous punch grafts also minimized to a great extent

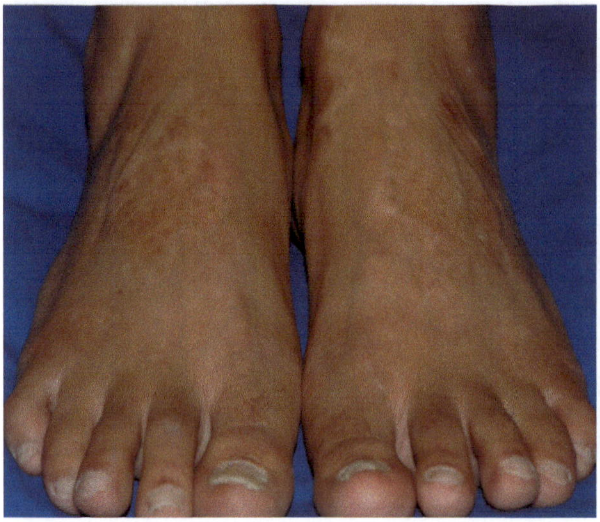

Figs. 17.2.13 Twenty-second month after microskin graft on residual lesion on the feet. Normal pigmentation with excellent color match

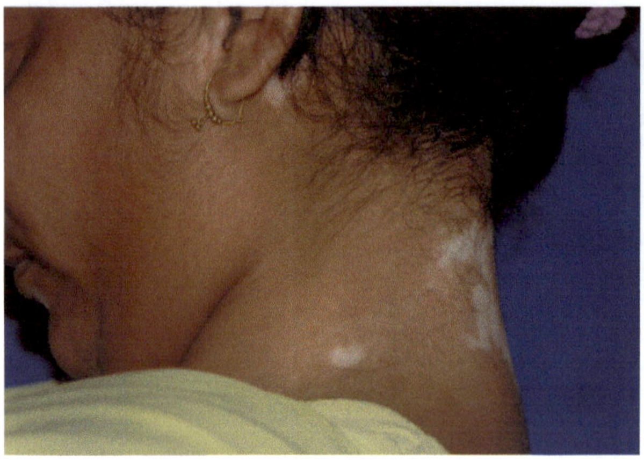

Figs. 17.2.14 Twenty-second post operative month – remarkable repigmentation on the left side of the neck and nape following oral mini pulse steroid therapy. The residual vitiliginous areas of the neck again need microskin grafting to complete the pigmentation

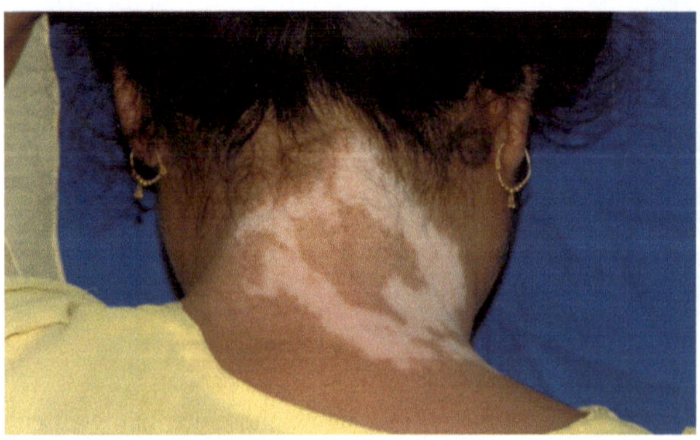

Figs. 17.2.15 Twenty-second post operative month – remarkable repigmentation of the neck and nape following oral mini pulse therapy

17.3 Case 3 (Segmental Vitiligo: Mini Punch Grafts vs. Microskin Grafts) (Figs. 17.3.1–17.3.11)

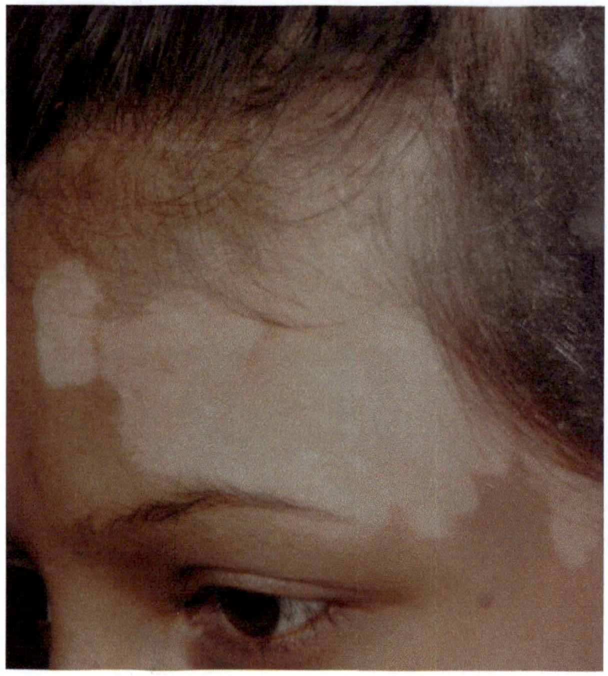

Fig. 17.3.1 A 18-year-old female with segmental vitiligo on the left side of the forehead before medical treatment

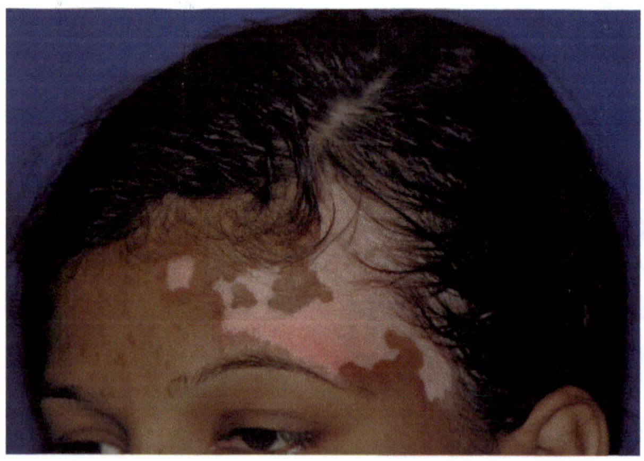

Fig. 17.3.2 Same patient with stable refractory segmental vitiligo on the left side of the forehead after medical treatment

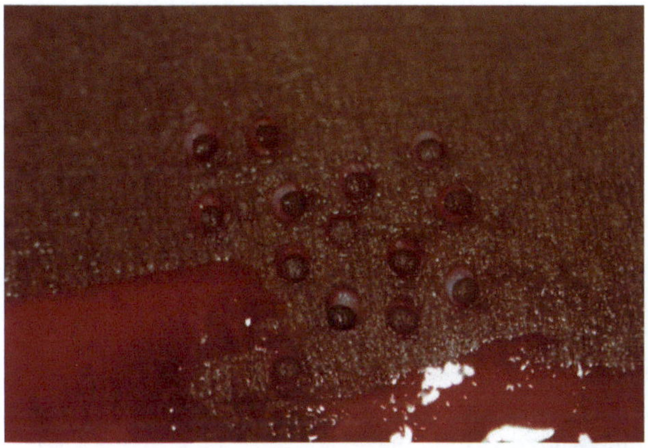

Fig. 17.3.3 Thin STSG graft is taken from the left gluteal fold with the help of Silver's miniature hand dermatome. Few mini punch grafts (1.2 mm) also removed from the same gluteal fold for comparative study (mini punch graft vs. microskin graft). Minipunch grafts were cut with help of 1.2 mm punch

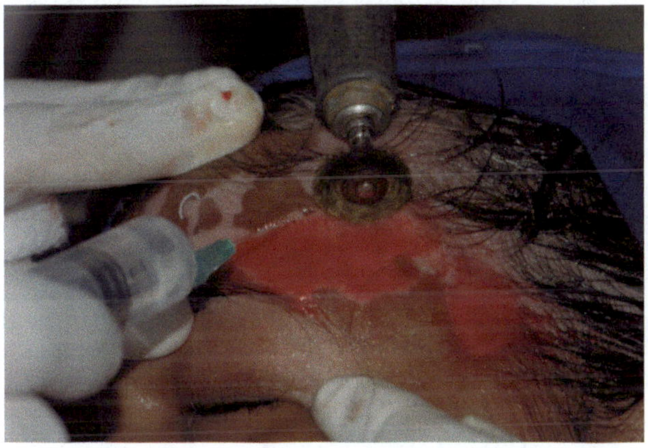

Fig. 17.3.4 Forehead vitiliginous area is superficially dermabraded with the help of the wire brush. During dermabrasion, the site is continuously kept wet with normal saline

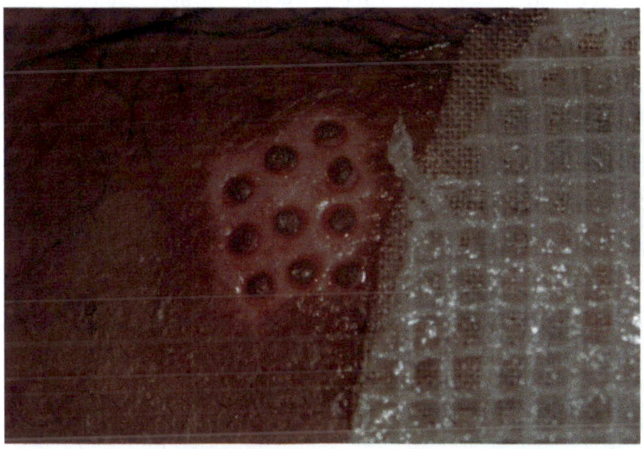

Fig. 17.3.5 A small white macule is selected on the mid forehead and 1 mm discs of skin are cut and removed. The 1.2 mm mini punch graft discs are transplanted at recipient site as shown

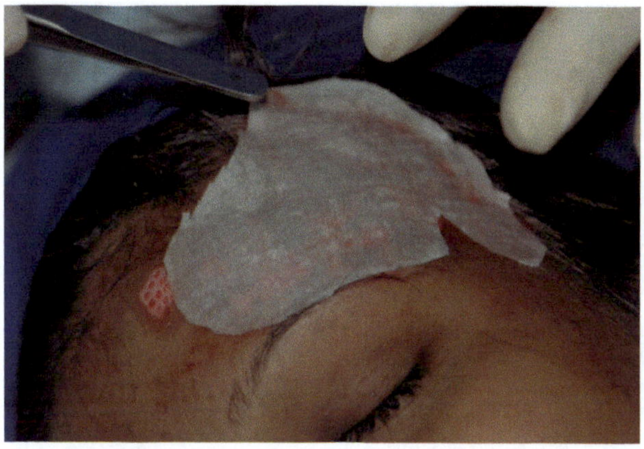

Fig. 17.3.6 The muslin sheet carrying the microskin grafts is applied over the dermabraded area of forehead. Minipunch grafts are also covered by dual layered tulle gras

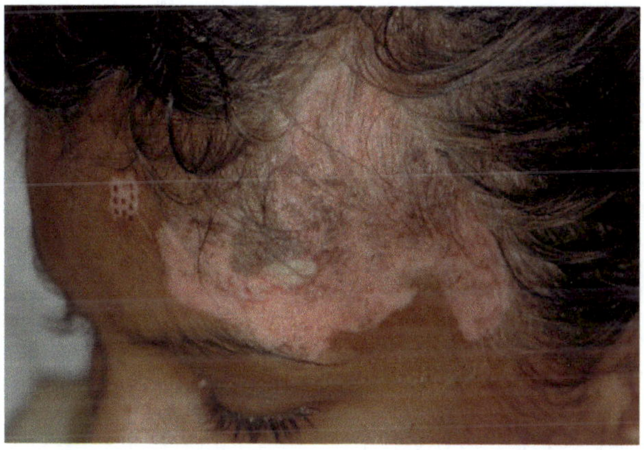

Fig. 17.3.7 Eleventh post operative day: microskin grafts accepted on the recipient site with a small area of infection just above the middle of the left eyebrow

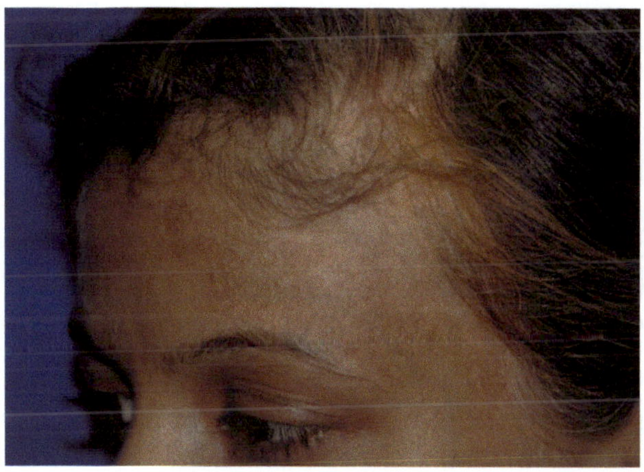

Fig. 17.3.8 Near normal pigmentation at 50th post operative day with microskin grafts

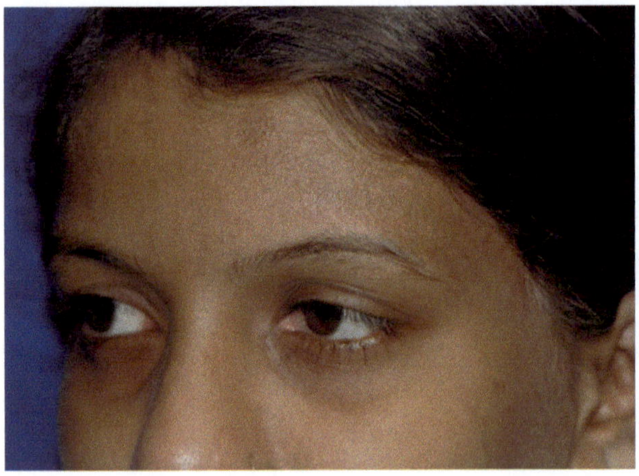

Fig. 17.3.9 Excellent natural color match with MSGs at 3.5 months. Cobblestoning effect at the site of MPGs is still visible at central forehead

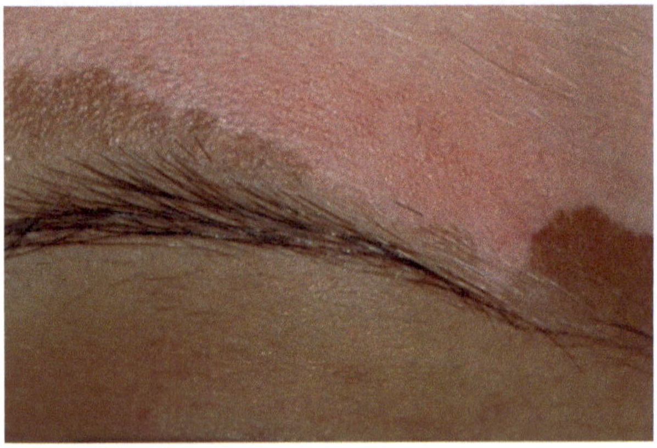

Fig. 17.3.10 Leukotrichia present in vitiliginous area above the left eyebrow

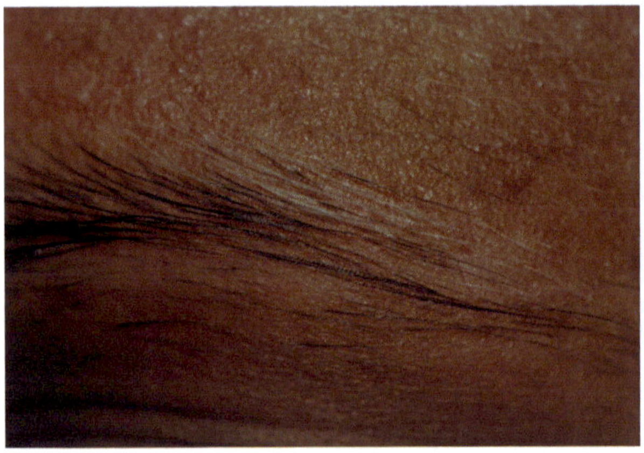

Fig. 17.3.11 White hair start becoming black at 3.5 months onward time

17.4 Case 4 (Acrofacial Vitiligo) (Figs. 17.4.1–17.4.6)

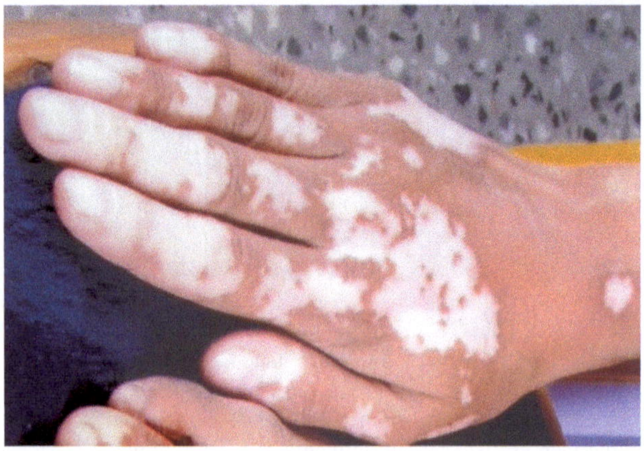

Fig. 17.4.1 Unstable vitiligo before medical treatment of right hand

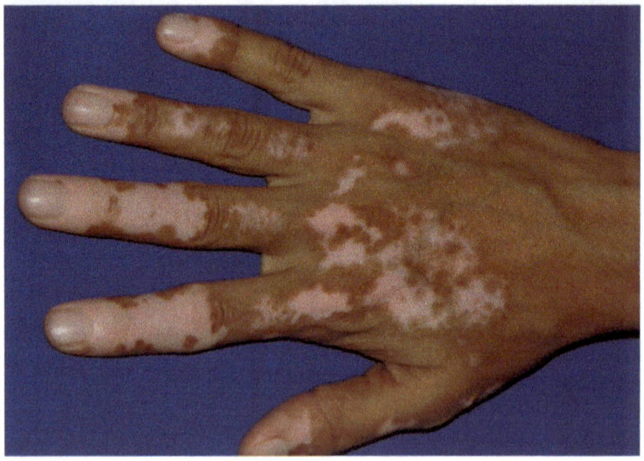

Fig. 17.4.2 Preoperative view of the right hand after 9 months of medical treatment. This refractory lesion planned for microskin grafting

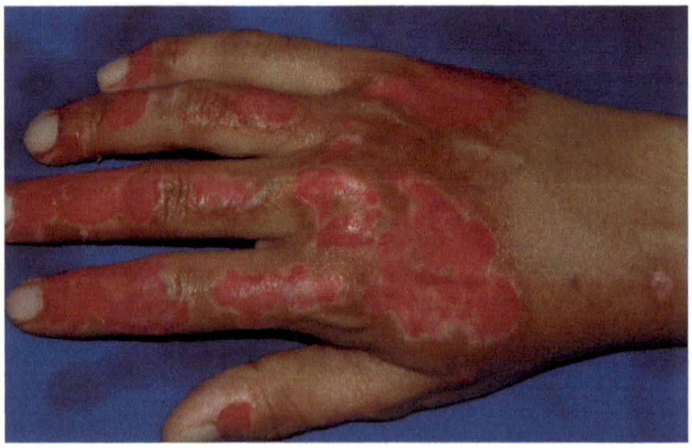

Fig. 17.4.3 Completion of dermabrasion of the hand

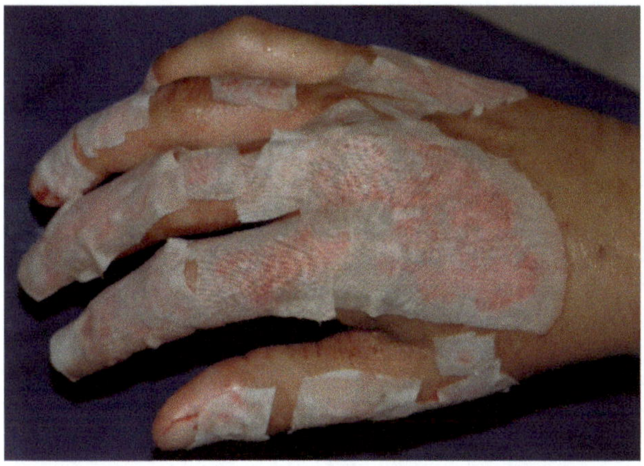

Fig. 17.4.4 Completion of microskin graft transplantation by floatation method. The muslin sheets applied carrying MSGs on its inner surface

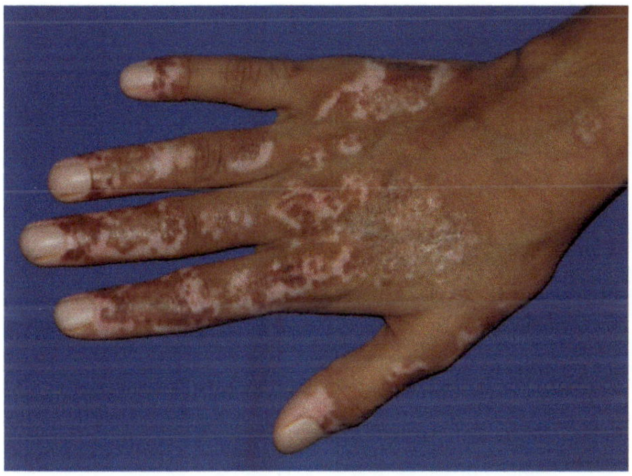

Fig. 17.4.5 Thirty-seventh post operative day: Fairly good pigmentation achieved. *Note*: Acral vitiliginous lesions take a long time (3–9 months) for complete repigmentation, following repopulation of vitiligo with melanocytes by repigmentary surgical therapies

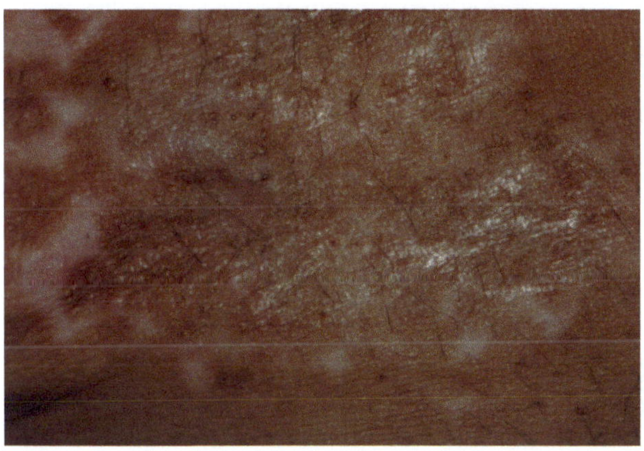

Fig. 17.4.6 Thirty-seventh post operative day: close up view of repigmentation on the dorsum of hand

17.5 Case 5 (Stable and Refractory Vitiligo Both Areola) (Figs. 17.5.1–17.5.14)

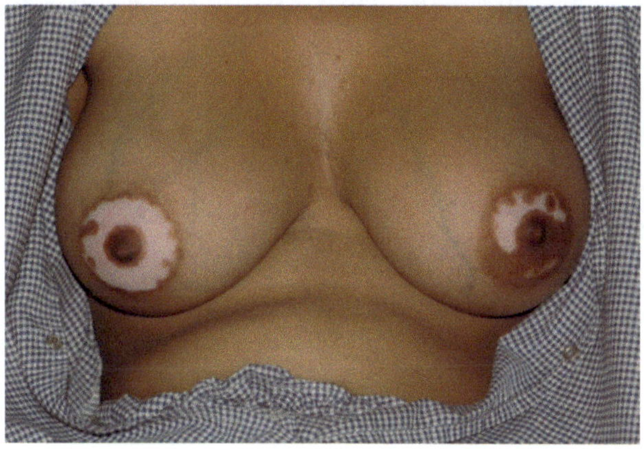

Fig. 17.5.1 A 20-year-old female having bilateral stable vitiligo of both areolas of the breast. She was on medical treatment for the last 6 months. The disease was not spreading and became refractory with medical treatment. Complete depigmentation of the right areola and the partial depigmentation of the left areola. She is now planned for microskin grafting

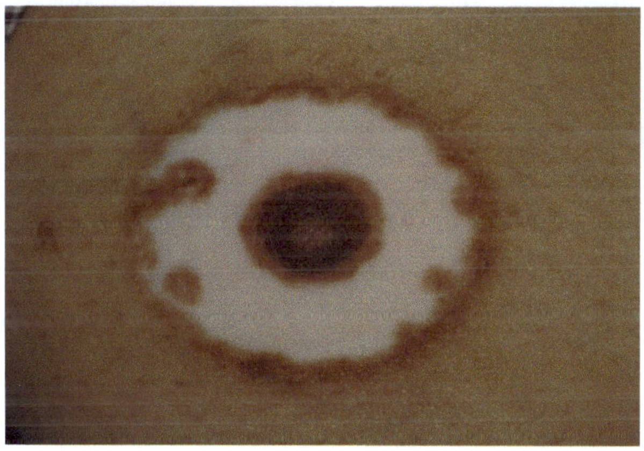

Fig. 17.5.2 Close up photograph of right areola showing vitiliginous area

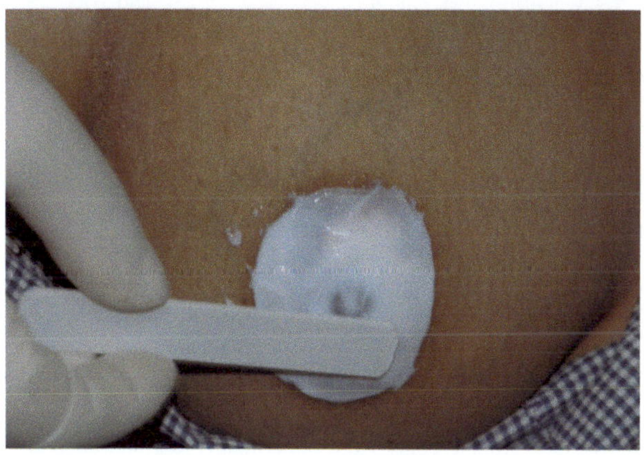

Fig. 17.5.3 Areola is covered by EMLA Cream with the help of spatula. Cream is applied in 2–3 mm thickness

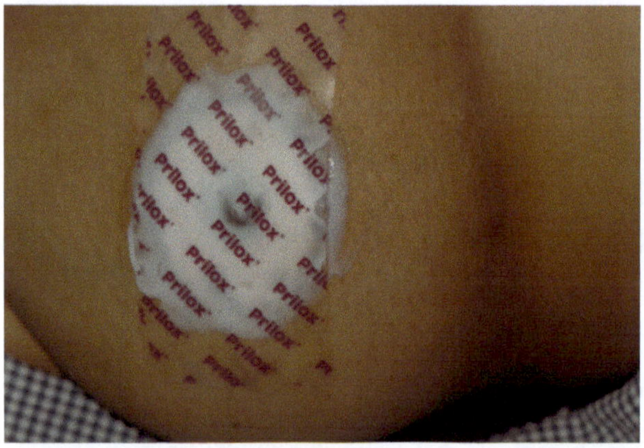

Fig. 17.5.4 Occlusive dressing is put on for 1.5 hours without compression

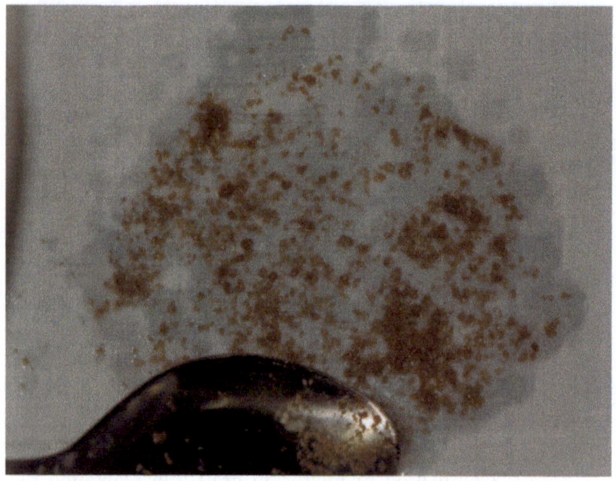

Fig. 17.5.7 Microskin grafts spread on the muslin sheet in a circular fashion according to the size of areola

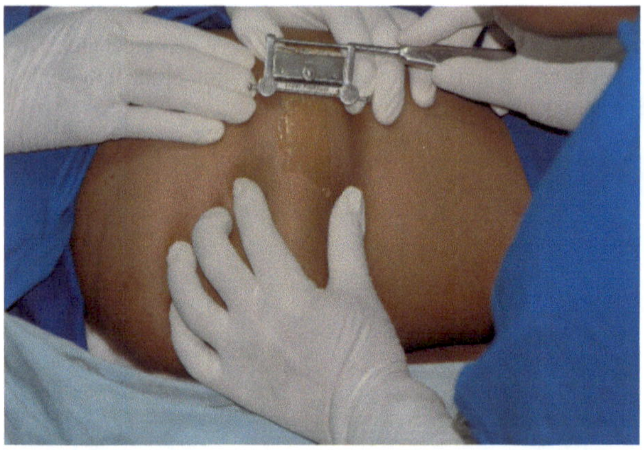

Fig. 17.5.5 Thin graft is harvested from the right gluteal fold with the help of Silver's miniature hand dermatome

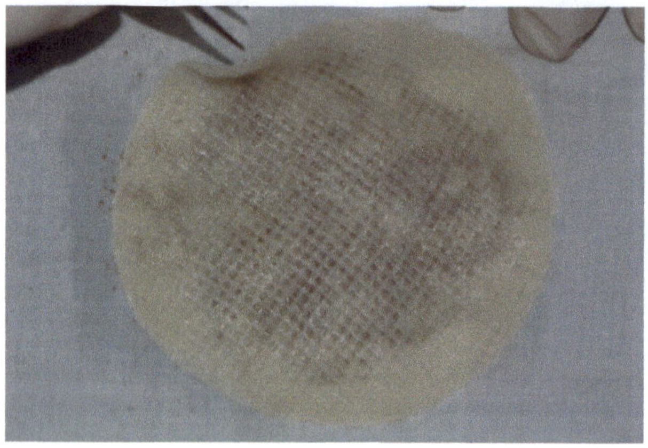

Fig. 17.5.8 Microskin graft turned over on circular white Vaseline impregnated tulle gras

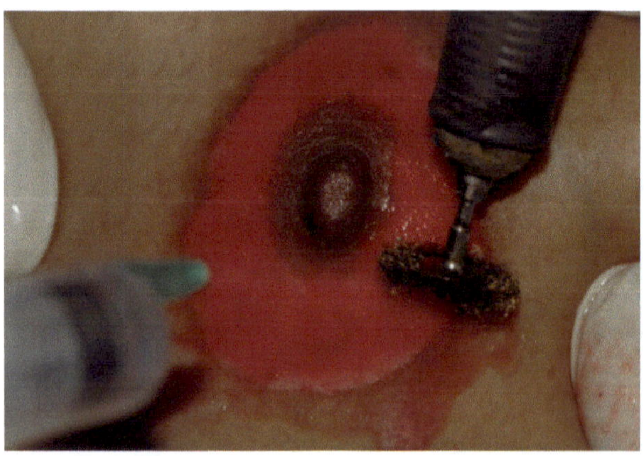

Fig. 17.5.6 Both areolas were superficially dermabraded by using wire brush as shown

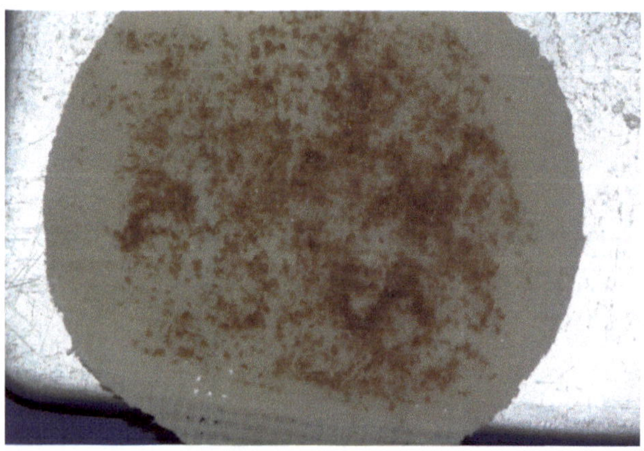

Fig. 17.5.9 Reversed microskin grafts on the circular tulle gras

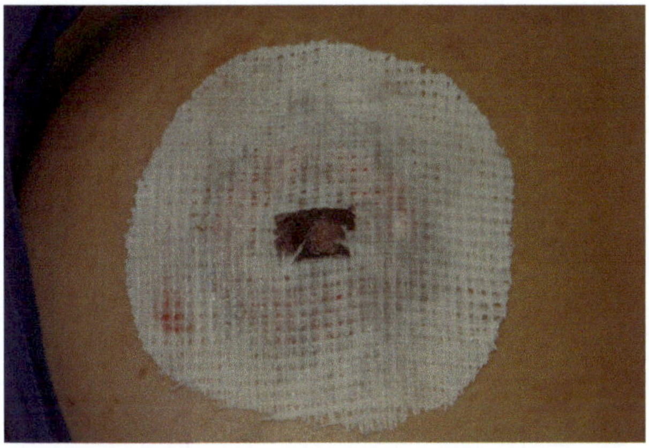

Fig. 17.5.10 Microskin grafts are transplanted on the areola and wet cotton is applied on tulle gras and finally covered by dry cotton gauge pads and fixed with hypo allergic tape

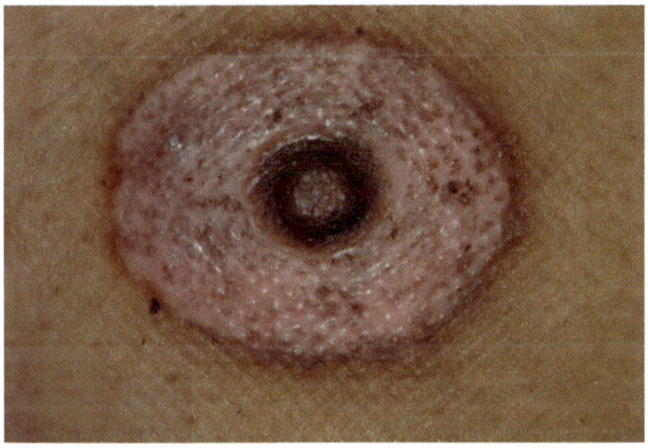

Fig. 17.5.11 Bandage removed on 10th day. Wound epithelized and grafts took well

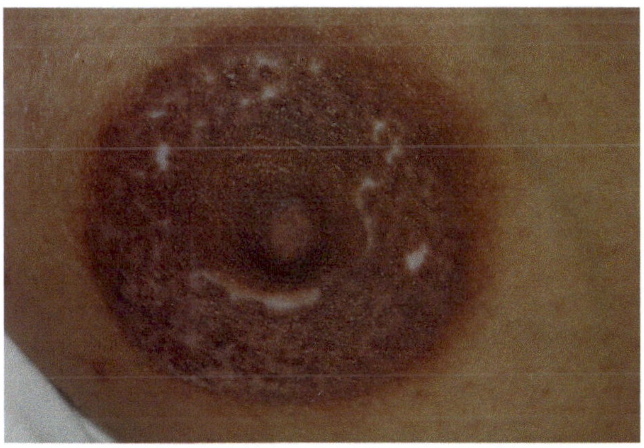

Fig. 17.5.12 Right areola after 21 days of microskin grafting

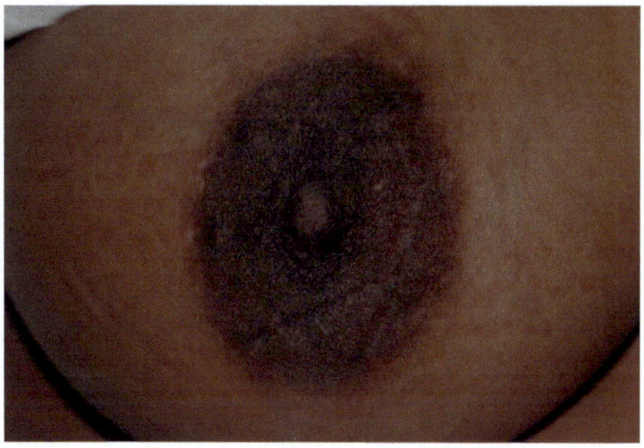

Fig. 17.5.13 Right areola after 108 days of microskin grafting

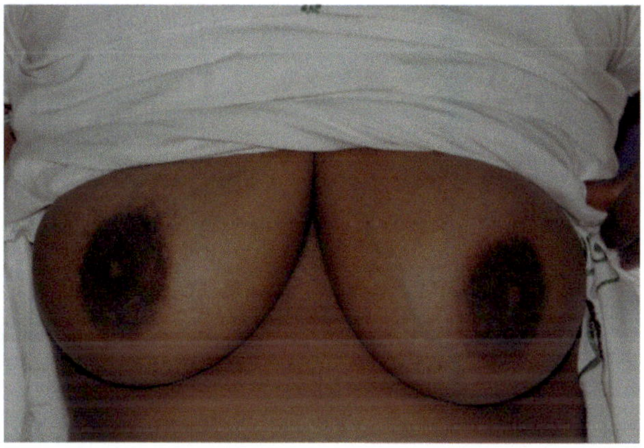

Fig. 17.5.14 After 108 days of microskin grafting. Perfectly normal pigmentation and color match

Microskin Grafting by Spraying Method in Extensive Vitiligo Management

18

Donor to recipient area ratio can be increased upto 1:15 by spraying method. For rapid and uniform pigmentation in 3–5 months time, the donor to recipient ratio should not be expanded beyond 1:8. Expansion beyond 1:15 will take longer time to repigment the area and some times residual lesions may need secondary surgery for repigmentation. During secondary surgery, the small residual intervening vitiliginous areas can be dermabraded carefully by diamond fraise to avoid abrasion of pigmented area. This is followed by the application of MSGs, which are floated in normal saline, with the help of sterilized dropper. The number of MSGs depends on the area of vitiliginous patch. For example an area of 0.25 cm^2 (0.5×0.5 cm) will ideally require only one MSG. Practically, I used to put at least 2–3 MSGs in such a small area due to uncertainty of orientation of graft.

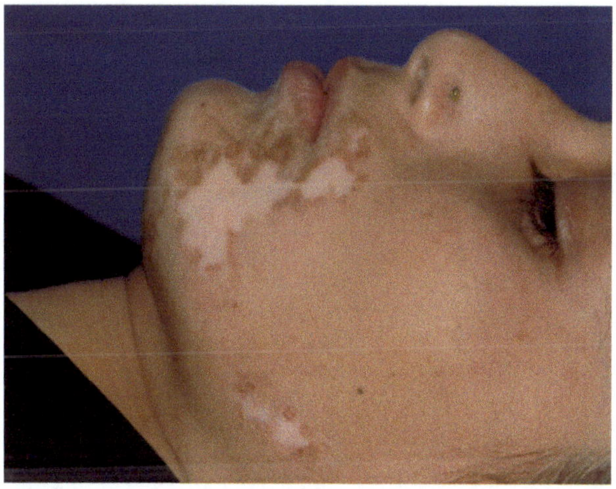

Fig. 18.1.1 Stable segmental vitiligo on left side of the face planned for microskin grafting. Local PUVASOL (Psoralen + UVA of solar origin) leads to recurrent blistering and scarring of the vitiliginous area on the cheek

18.1 Case 1 (Stable Segmental Vitiligo-Cheek)

A 20-year-old female patient had vitiligo on her right cheek for the last 13 years. She was treated by various herbs and local PUVASOL (Psoralen plus ultra violet-A of solar origin). Chronic treatment by various local applications led to scarring in white macule. This stable and refractory lesion was planned for microskin grafting (Figs. 18.1.1–18.1.7).

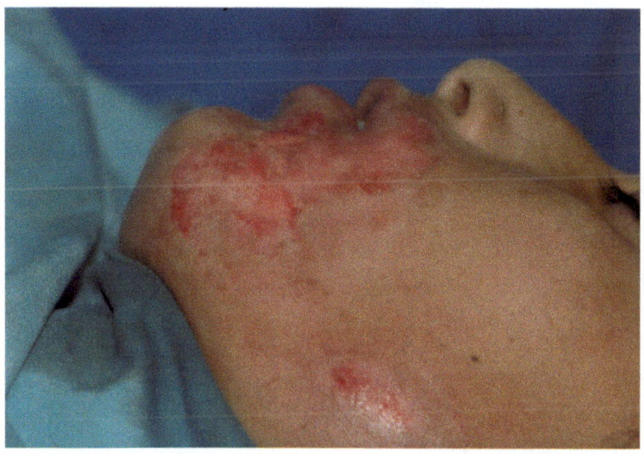

Fig. 18.1.2 Dermabrasion completed with diamond fraise

D. K. Gupta, *Microskin Grafting for Vitiligo*,
DOI: 10.1007/978-1-84882-605-2_18, © Springer Science + Business Media B.V. 2009

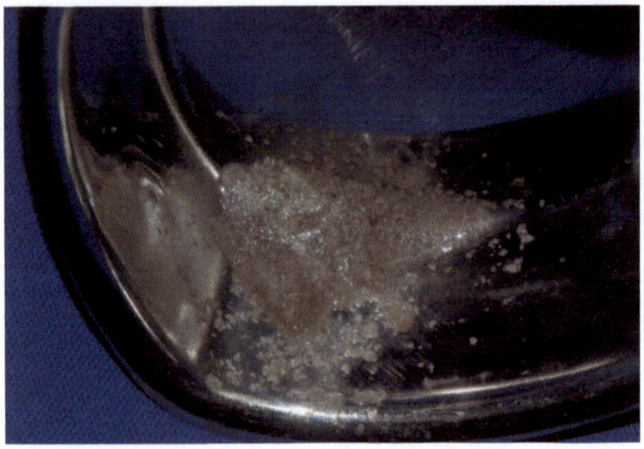

Fig. 18.1.3 Ultra thin skin graft transformed into microskin grafts (MSGs) by scissor

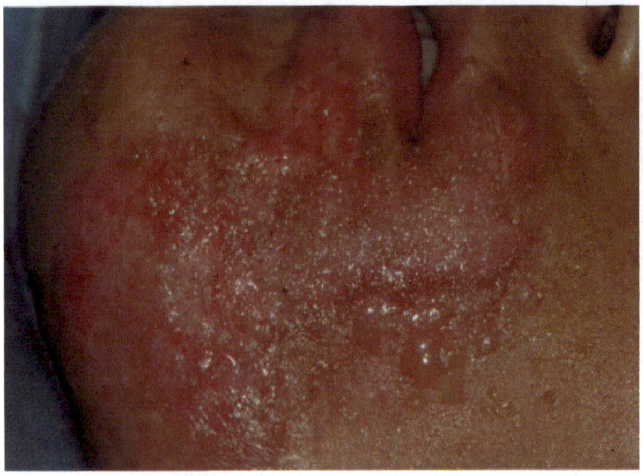

Fig. 18.1.4 Close up view of directly sprayed MSGs on dermabraded area of the face

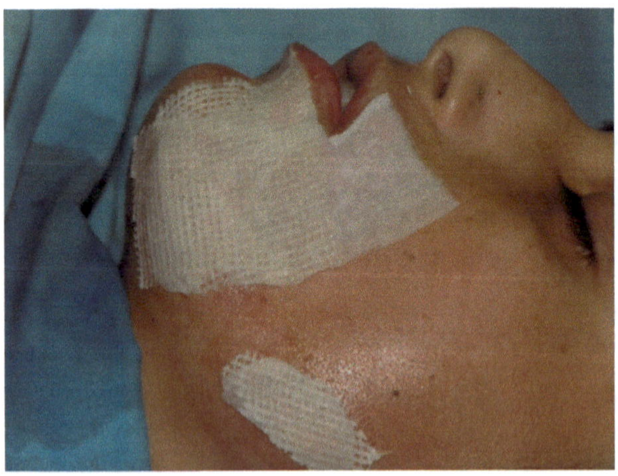

Fig. 18.1.5 Wet muslin sheet and Vaseline tulle gras applied over MSGs

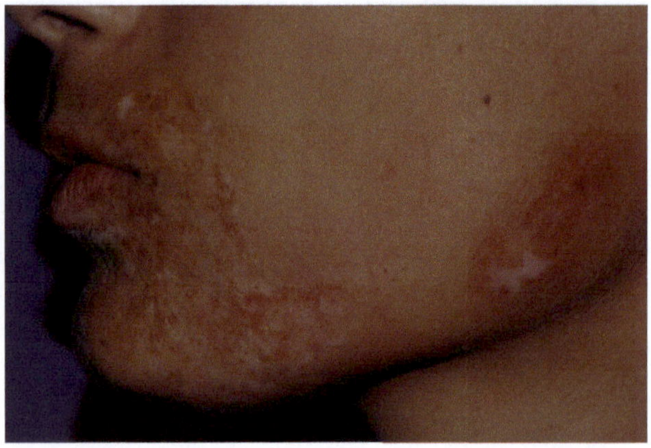

Fig. 18.1.6 Pigmentation achieved at 56th day. Scarring following PUVASOL is quite obvious now

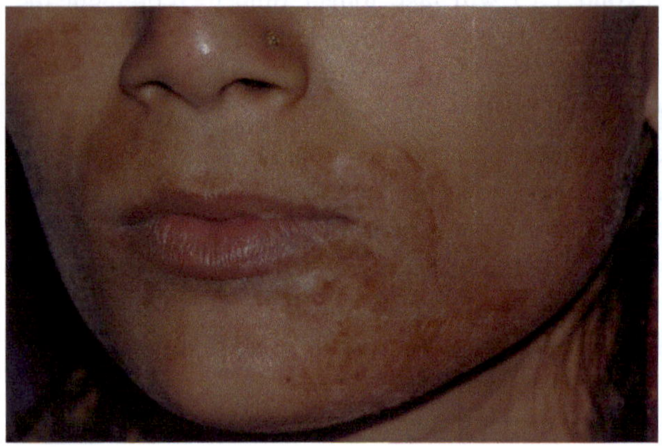

Fig. 18.1.7 Pigmentation achieved at 71days

18.2 Case 2 (Vitiligo Vulgaris)

A 20-year-old female patient was kept on trioxsalen and steroid oral mini pulse (OMP) therapy. In about 3 months time progression of the disease stopped and new pigmentation started. After having observed the stability of the disease for 1 year, she was planned for microskin grafting. She had white macules all over her body e.g. eyelids, pinna, nape, wrist, elbows, right thigh, both knees, both legs, both ankles and both feet.

18.2.1 First Microskin Graft Operation

The first operation was performed on superolateral aspect of right knee, leg and ankle (Figs. 18.2.1.1–18.2.1.19)

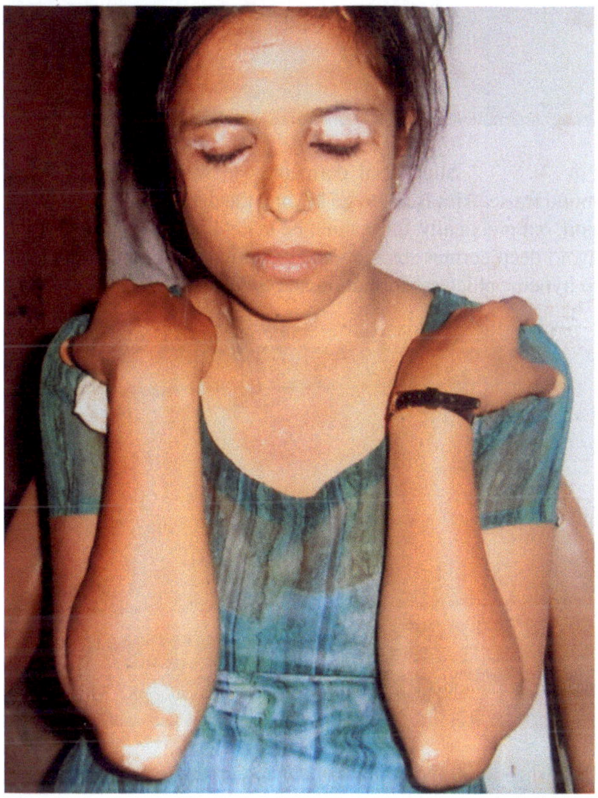

Fig. 18.2.1.1 A case of vitiligo vulgaris (before medical treatment). She had white macules all over her body, e.g., eyelids, pinna, nape, wrist, elbows, right thigh, both knees, both legs, both ankles and both feet

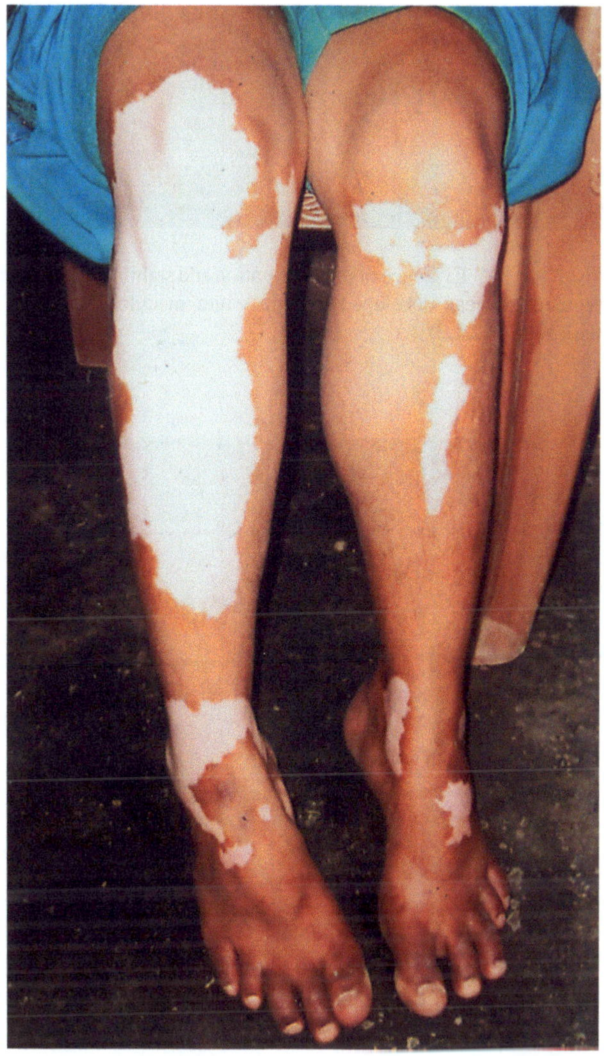

Fig. 18.2.1.2 Same case of vitiligo vulgaris (before medical treatment). She had white macules over her right thigh, both knees, both legs, both ankles and both feet

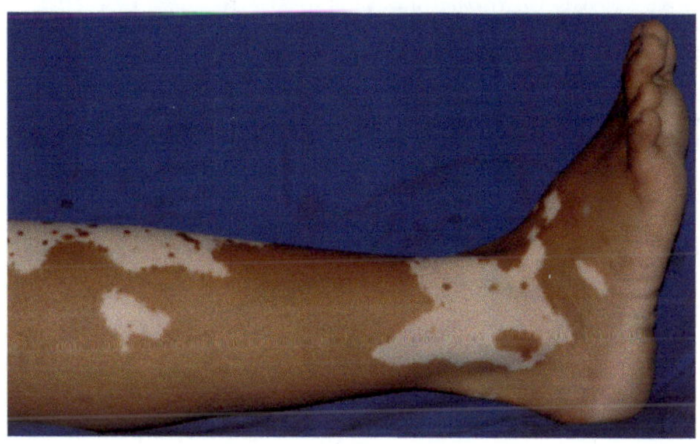

Fig. 18.2.1.3 Evidence of repigmentation and stability. Multiple pigmented areas developed in pure white macules (compare with **Fig 18.2.1.2**)

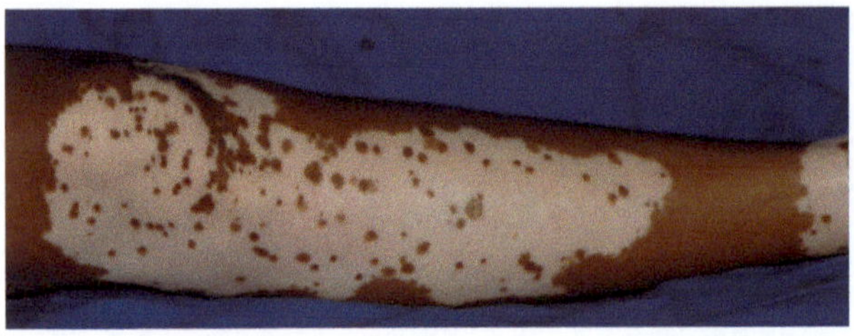

Fig. 18.2.1.4 Evidence of repigmentation and stability. Multiple pigmented areas developed in pure white macules (compare with **Fig. 18.2.1.2**)

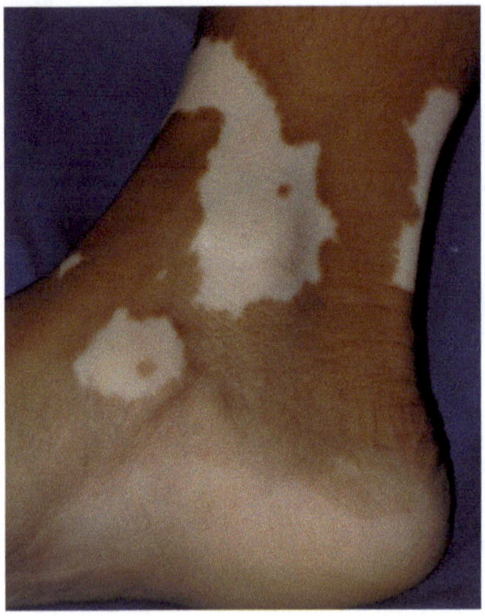

Fig. 18.2.1.5 Evidence of repigmentation and stability. Multiple pigmented areas developed in pure white macules

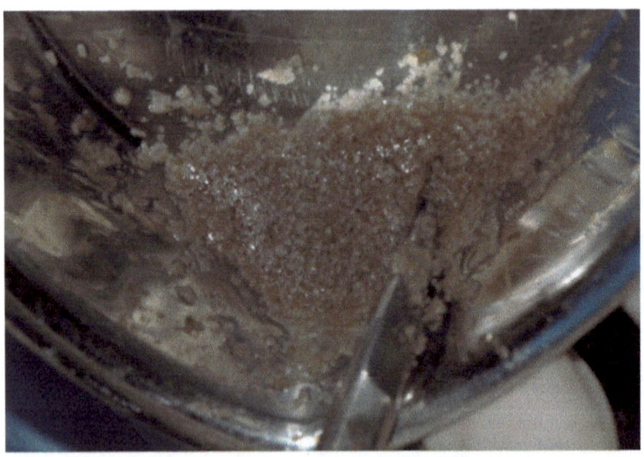

Fig. 18.2.1.6 While the surgeon performs the dermabrasion, an assistant prepares the microskin grafts with the help of scissor. Ultra thin or thin STSG is kept in a tray with a few drops of normal saline. Assistant then cuts this skin sheet into very small skin particles which are mostly between 0.2 and 0.5 mm in size. This can be easily accomplished in 10–15 minutes time. These small skin particles or pieces practically transforms into a thick paste

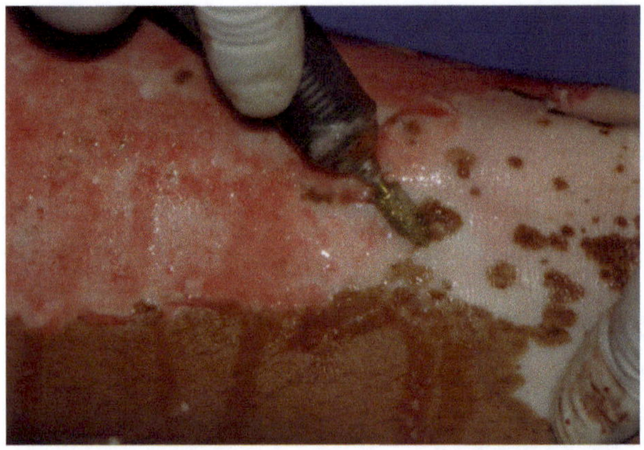

Fig. 18.2.1.7 Superficial dermabrasion with the help of diamond fraise. Aim is not to go beyond the dermo-epidermal junction, but practically, this cannot be maintained. Instead carefully avoid deep dermal abrasion and gauging because this may lead to hypertrophic scar formation and more chances of infection

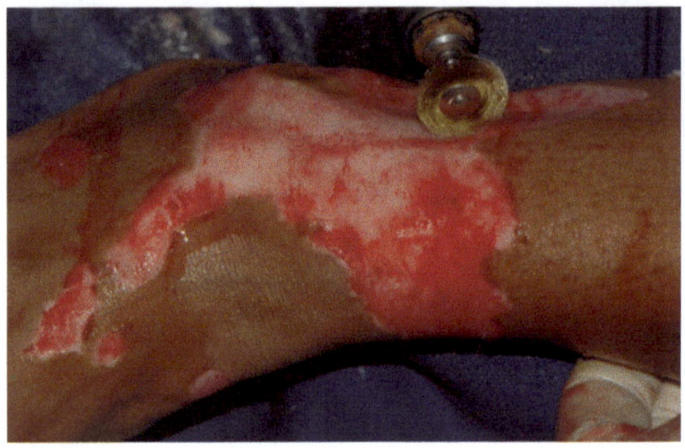

Fig. 18.2.1.8 Superficial dermabrasion is demonstrated by wire brush. Wire brush does dermabrasion by microlacerations. Of course, using wire brush requires more skilful steady hand than using diamond fraise. A beginner should learn dermabrasion by using diamond fraise

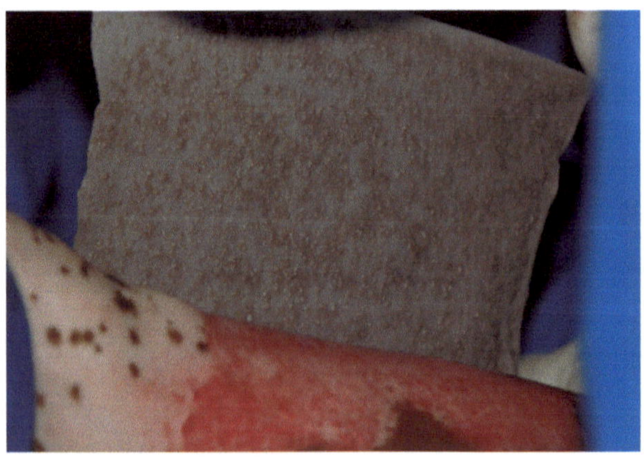

Fig. 18.2.1.9 The muslin cloth carrying scattered microskin grafts on one of its surface is applied over the dermabraded area of the leg as demonstrated

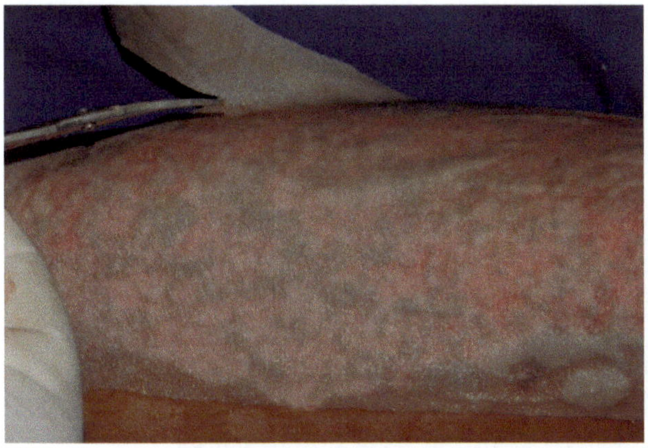

Fig. 18.2.1.10 The redundant muslin sheet is excised and kept to be applied on other dermabraded area

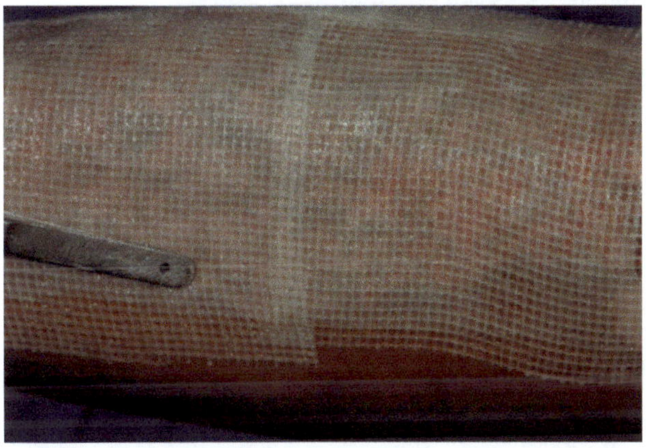

Fig. 18.2.1.11 Vaseline impregnated tulle gras is applied over the muslin sheet and gently ironed with the back of forceps or spatula, so that all the microskin grafts come in contact with abraded areas. The Vaseline of the tulle gras percolates the muslin sheet so that this can be easily separated out during dressing removal

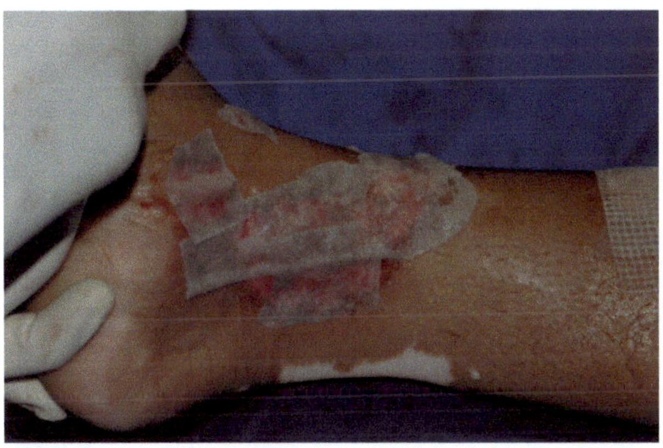

Fig. 18.2.1.12 Dermabraded vitiliginous area of the ankle covered by small cut pieces of muslin sheet that carries scattered microskin grafts on one of its side. These cut muslin pieces are leftovers of the large sheets used to cover large dermabraded areas

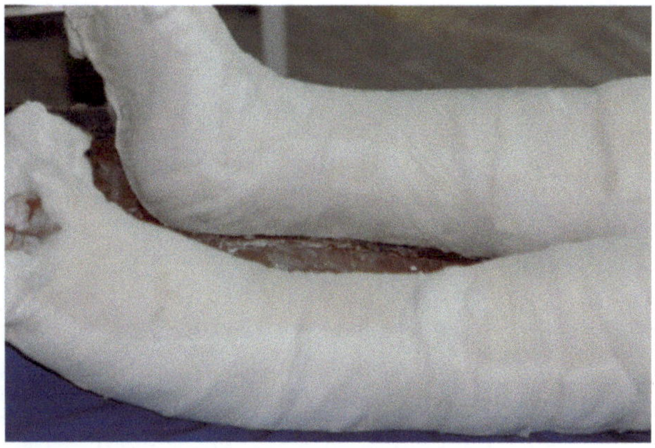

Fig. 18.2.1.13 Normal saline wet muslin sheets are covered by white vaseline impregnated tulle gras, cotton pads and finally splinted to avoid shearing movements and dislodgement of the MSGs

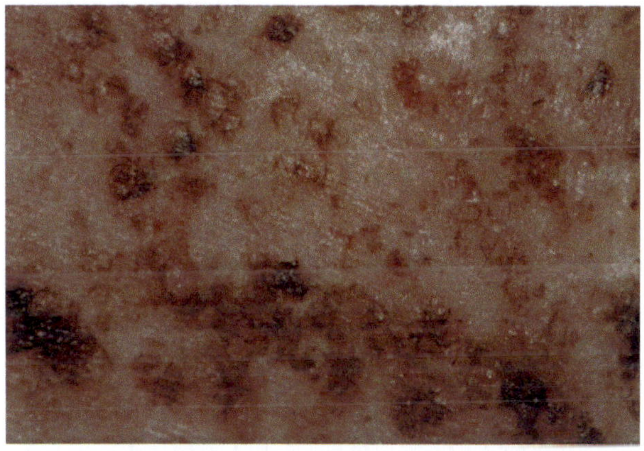

Fig. 18.2.1.14 Eighth post operative day: close up view of microskin graft "take"

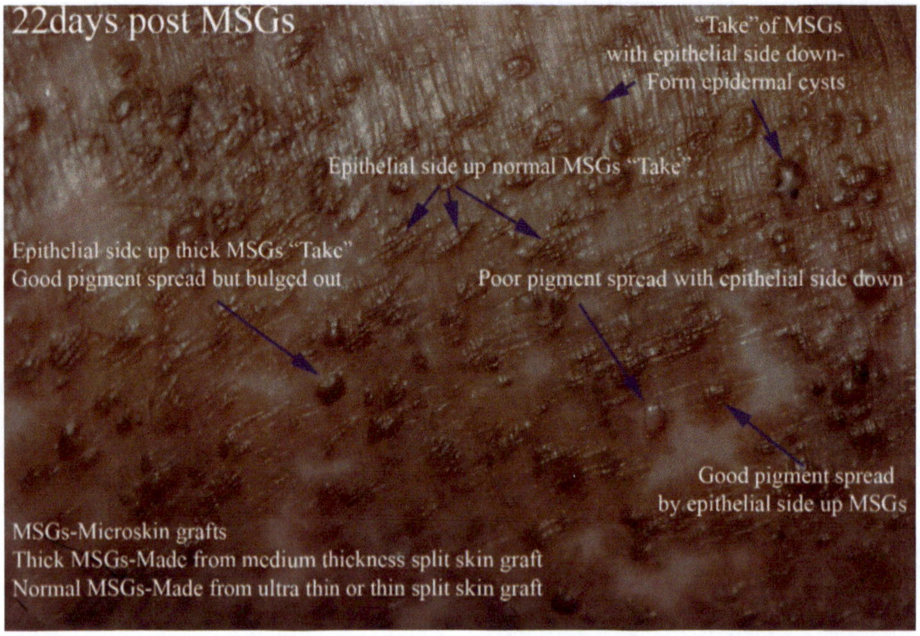

Fig. 18.2.1.15 Twenty-second post operative day: close up photograph of the right leg. This photograph shows the "take" of epithelial side up thin, little thicker and epithelial side down (reversed) microskin grafts. Thin and normally oriented microskin grafts take well and remain shriveled and flat on the recipient area. Good amount of rapid repigmentation is achieved by these grafts. Little thicker grafts also take but remain bulged and produce the same amount of pigmentation as the thinner one. Epithelial side down microskin grafts also "take" but to a little lesser extent. These may get vascularized from its margin. These remain bulged due to formation of epidermal cysts which get ruptured in due coarse of time. Pigment spread is rather slow from these reversed microskin grafts. Underneath these reversed grafts the skin remains little white in the centre. The minor cobblestone produced by thicker and reversed microskin grafts. This cobblestone effect disappears in a few months

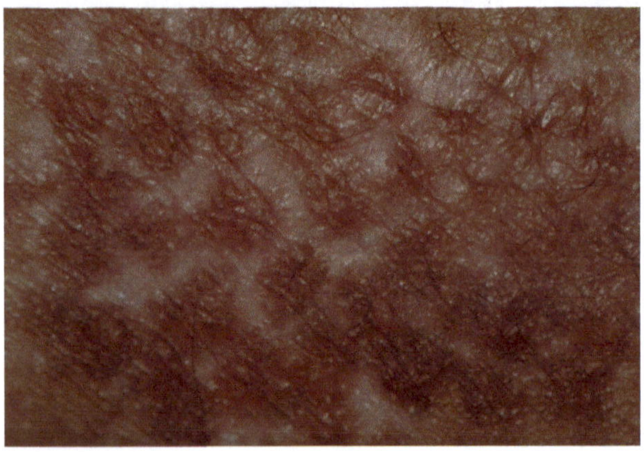

Fig. 18.2.1.16 Twenty-second day photograph of the donor area shows perifollicular pigmentation. After graft removal, the donor area becomes whitish due to exposed dermis

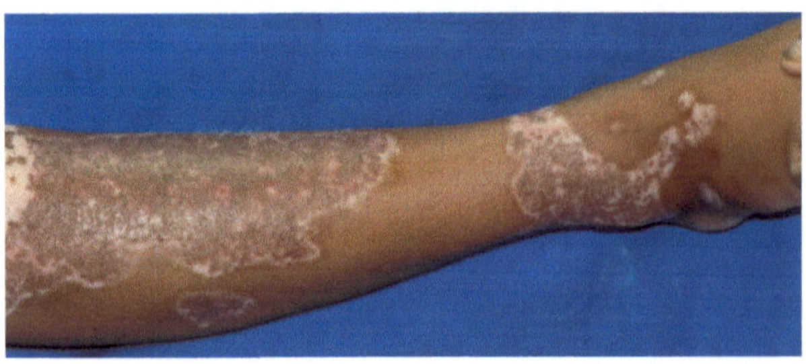

Fig. 18.2.1.17 Twenty-second post operative day: remarkable pigmentation

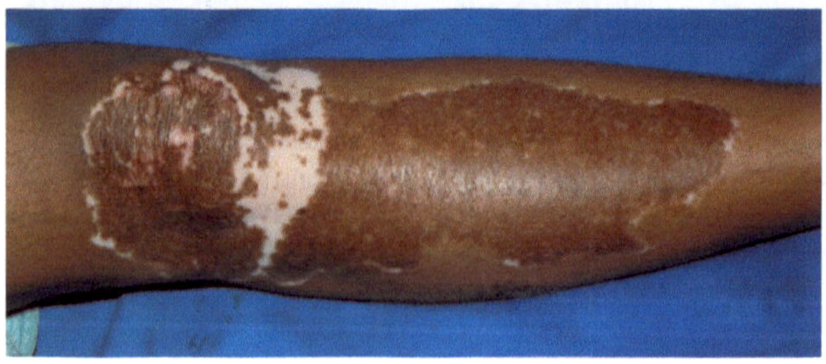

Fig. 18.2.1.18 Sixty-third post operative day: treated area shows excellent pigmentation. The peripheral area also starts mixing with the normal skin. At this time, most of the hair roots are white except a few. Please note that small infrapatellar area was not treated in first Microskin graft operation

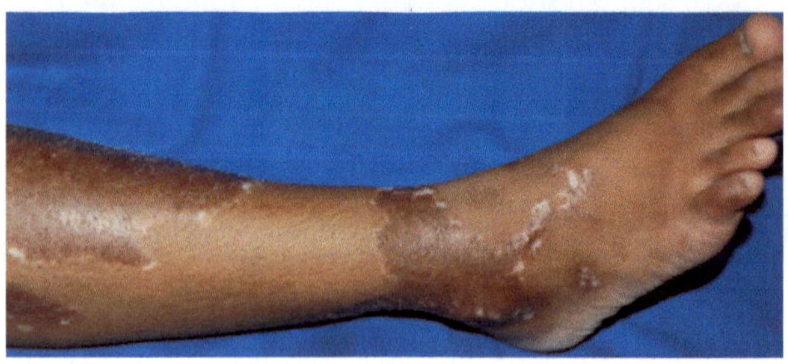

Fig. 18.2.1.19 Sixty-third post operative day: except a few scattered white area (3–12 mm), the ankle region pigmented well. The pigmented area is little darker than the surrounding skin. The natural color match may take another few months

18.2.2 Second Microskin Graft Operation Performed in the Same Patient After 63 Days

Second microskin graft operation was performed 63 days after the first operation to repigment – the untreated left knee, leg, foot, back of right elbow, ankle and right infrapatellar area. The ultra thin split thickness skin graft was removed from the left thigh. Part of this graft sheet was preserved in the refrigerator at 4°C for repigmentation of nape, eyelids, both pinna and side of neck, at the 5th day of second operation. Make sure that the stability of the disease is the one and the only important parameter for the selection of the patient, for surgery to be successful (Figs 18.2.2.1-18.2.2.7).

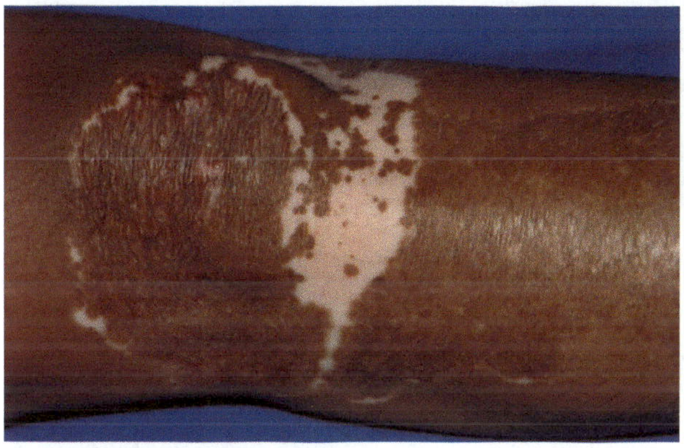

Fig. 18.2.2.1 The area below the patella of knee was not previously microskin grafted, remained as such and planned in this second stage surgery for repigmentation

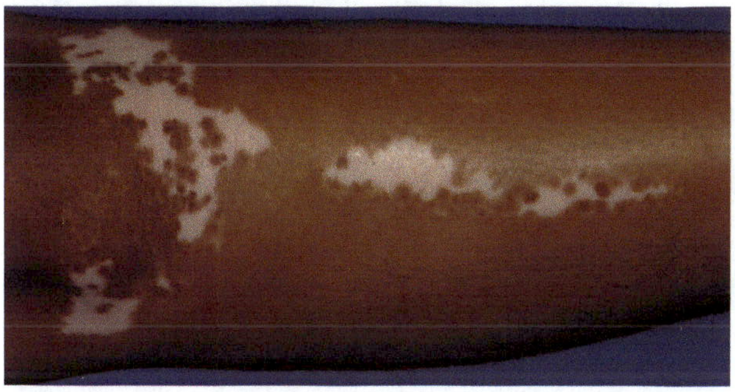

Fig. 18.2.2.2 Stable Vitiligo on Front of left knee and leg

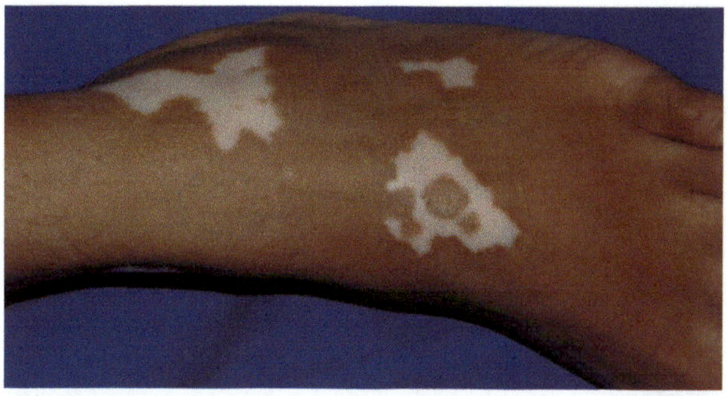

Fig. 18.2.2.3 Stable Vitiligo on front and lateral side of left ankle

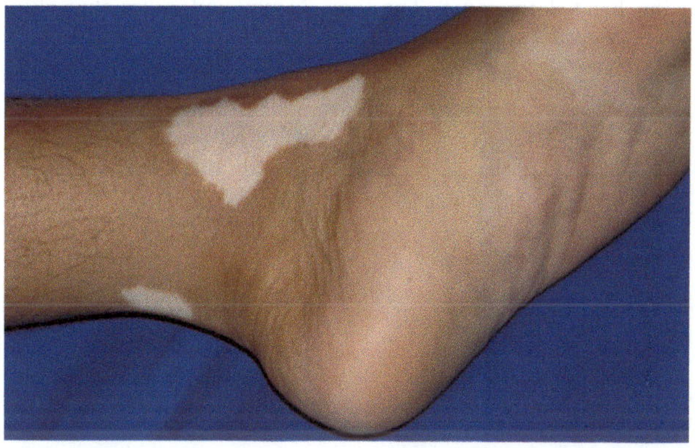

Fig. 18.2.2.4 Stable Vitiligo on medial side and back of left ankle

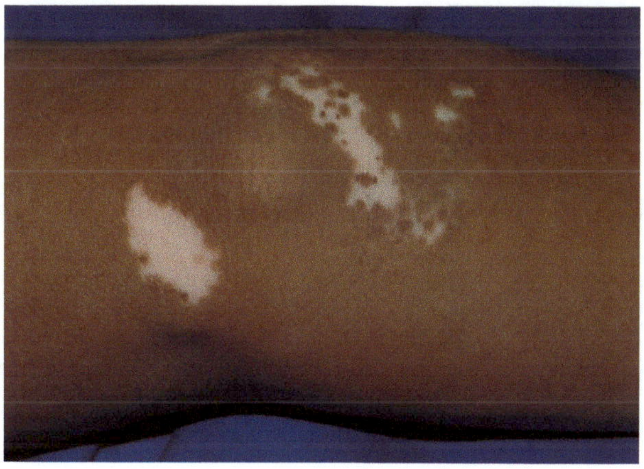

Fig. 18.2.2.5 Stable Vitiligo on back of right elbow

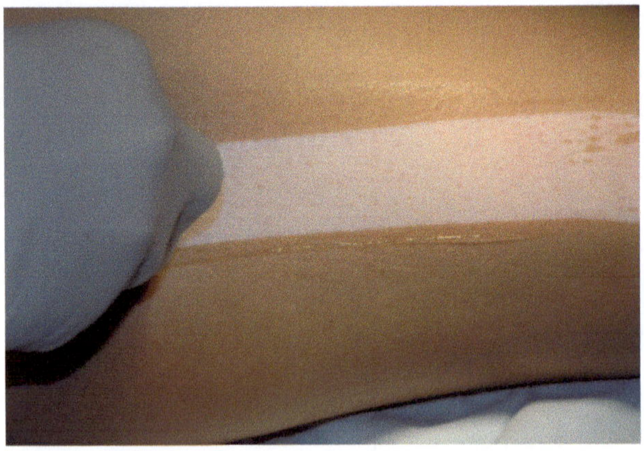

Fig. 18.2.2.6 Graft harvesting from the thigh. This photograph depicts the graft harvesting from the anterior aspect of the thigh using hand dermatome. The long 34 mm wide ultra thin skin strip is removed from the thigh

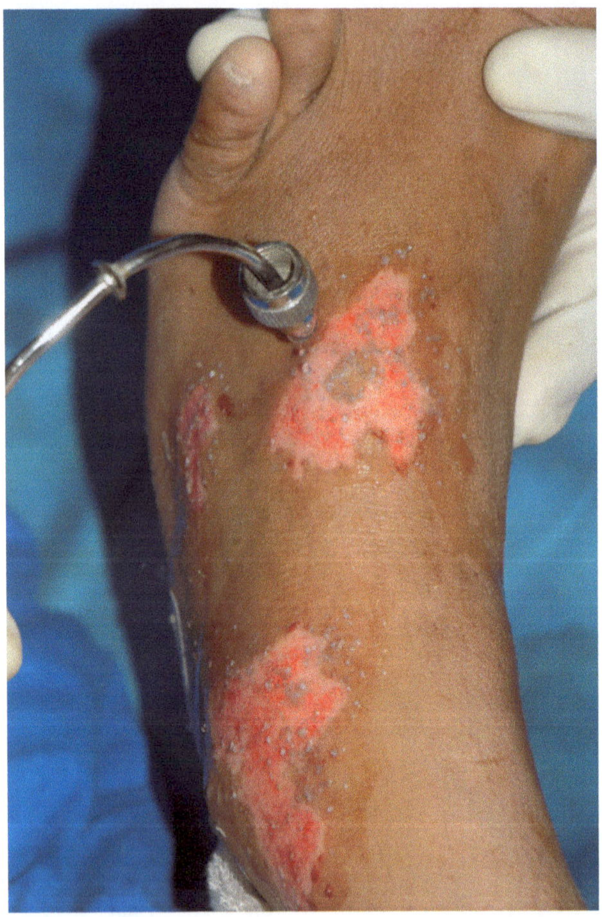

Fig. 18.2.2.7 Microskin graft is being sprayed with the help of a spraying device on vitiliginous areas of the left foot and the ankle. The spraying increases the expansion ratio of donor to recipient area from 1:5 to 1:15. Even one can go up to 1:40. But at this expansion ratio (1:40) the repigmentation takes little more time. Thus, I kept 1:5–1:10 expansion ratio ideal for repigmentation within the optimum time. Scattered skin particles away from the abraded areas are collected back on the peripheral part of the vitiliginous areas that is supposed to be resistant and the last to pigment

18.2.3 Third Microskin Graft Operation done on fifth day of second operation

Five days old graft sheet (preserved in the refrigerator at 4°C) was used for repigmentation of nape,eyelids, both pinna and side of neck, at the 5th day of second operation (Figs. 18.2.3.1-18.2.3.15).

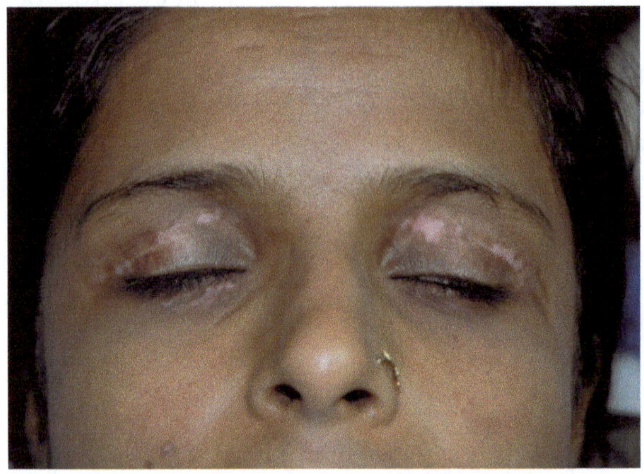

Fig. 18.2.3.1 Vitiligo on both upper and lower eyelids

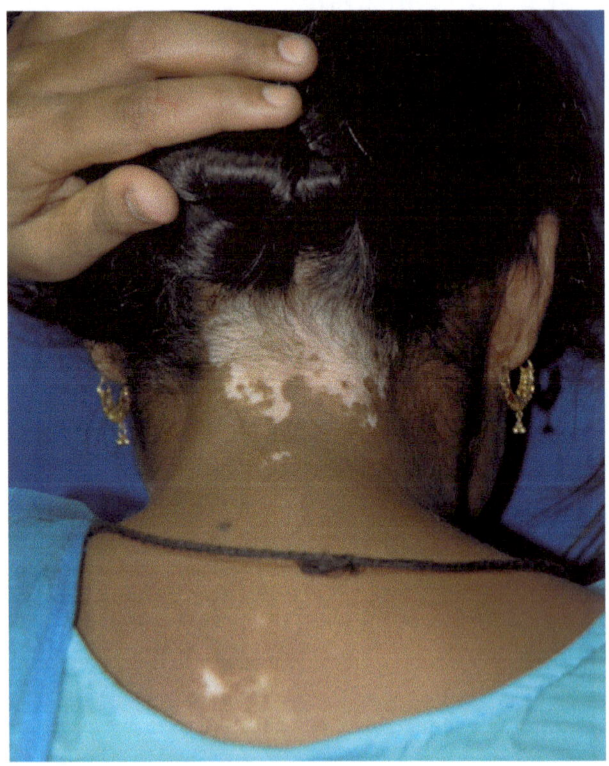

Fig. 18.2.3.2 Vitiligo on the nape and back of the upper part of the chest

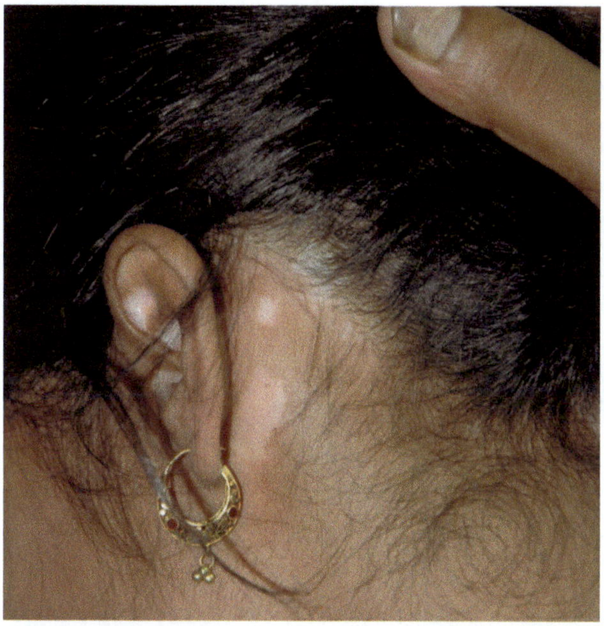

Fig. 18.2.3.3 Vitiligo left pinna and left post auricular area

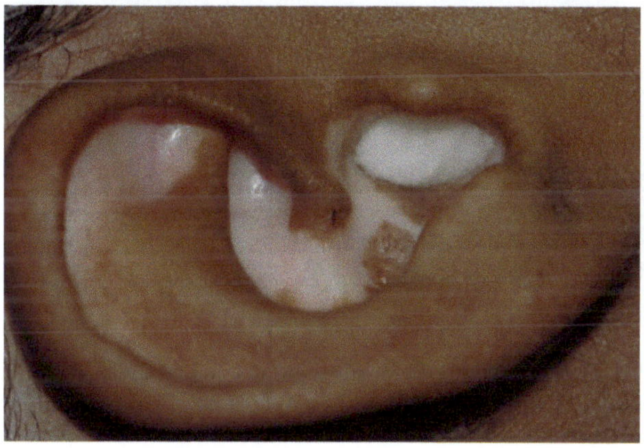

Fig. 18.2.3.4 Vitiligo right Pinna – close up view

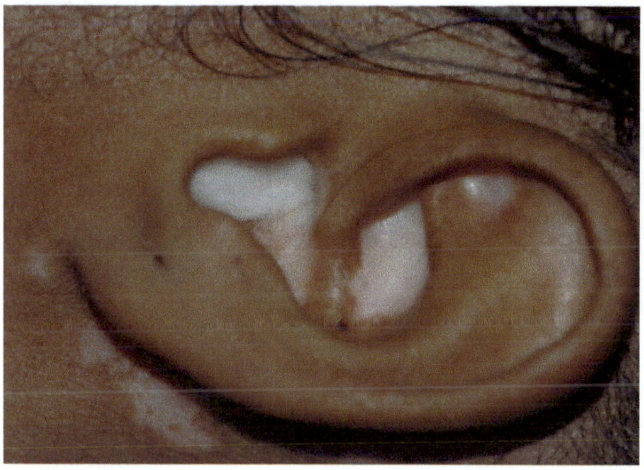

Fig. 18.2.3.5 Vitiligo left Pinna – close up view

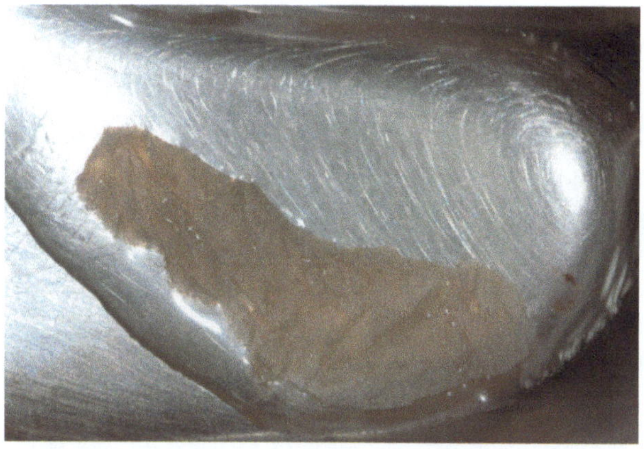

Fig. 18.2.3.6 Five days old preserved (kept at 4°C in refrigerator) ultra thin split thickness skin graft (STSG-UT)

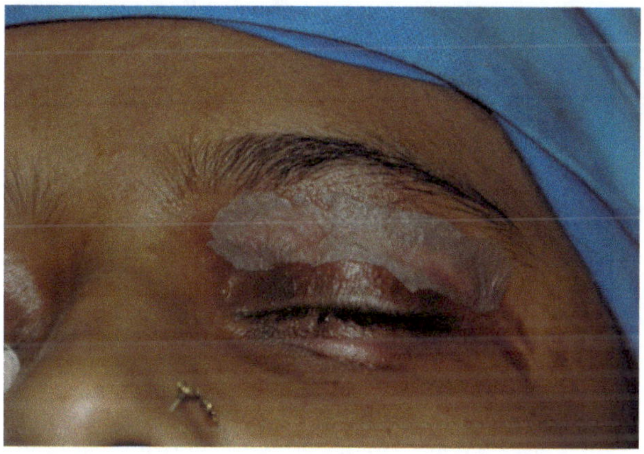

Fig. 18.2.3.7 A strip of STSG-UT spread on the dermabraded left upper eyelid and fixed to the skin of the eyelid by fine sutures

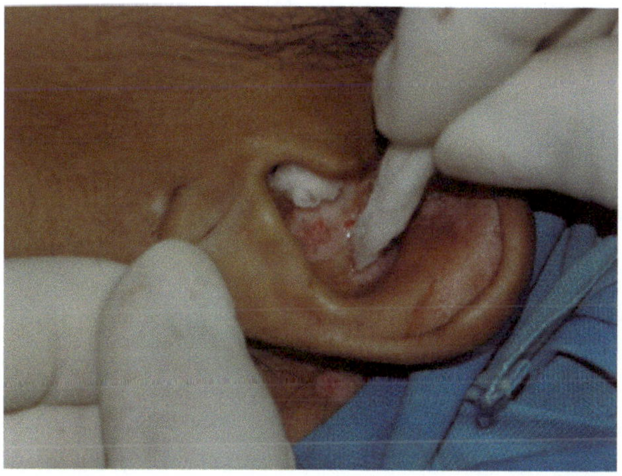

Fig. 18.2.3.8 Excess amount of normal saline is removed by the capillary action of cotton wick from deepest part of conchal area, after spraying microskin grafts

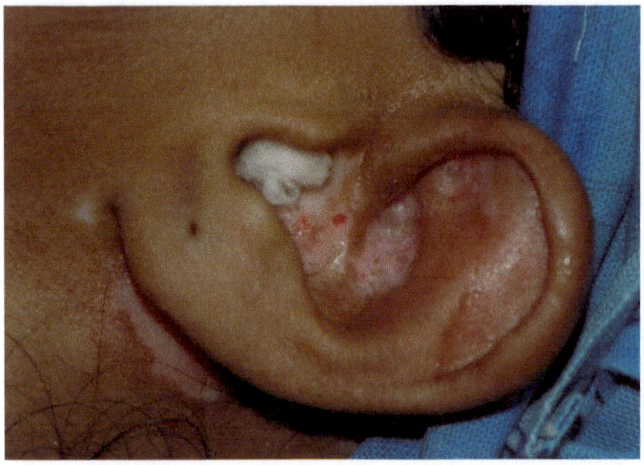

Fig. 18.2.3.9 Microskin grafts transplanted on the dermabraded areas of left pinna

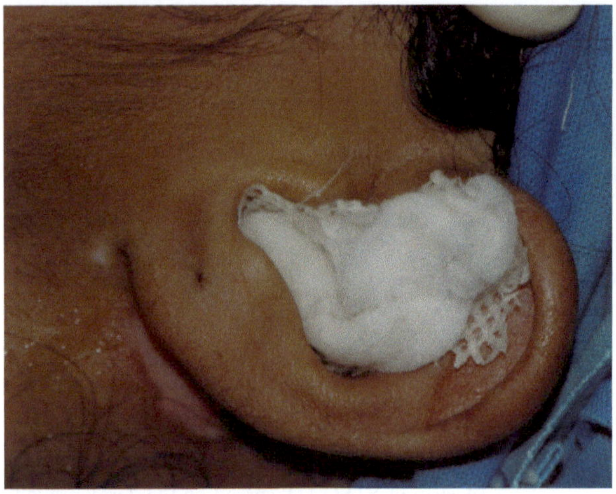

Fig. 18.2.3.10 Microskin grafts covered by Vaseline tulle gras. Concha and scapha of pinna is packed by wet cotton as shown

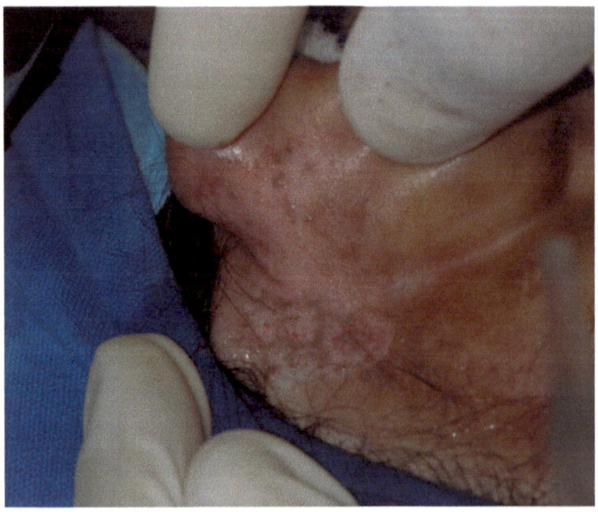

Fig. 18.2.3.11 Microskin grafting of the back side of the right pinna and post auricular area

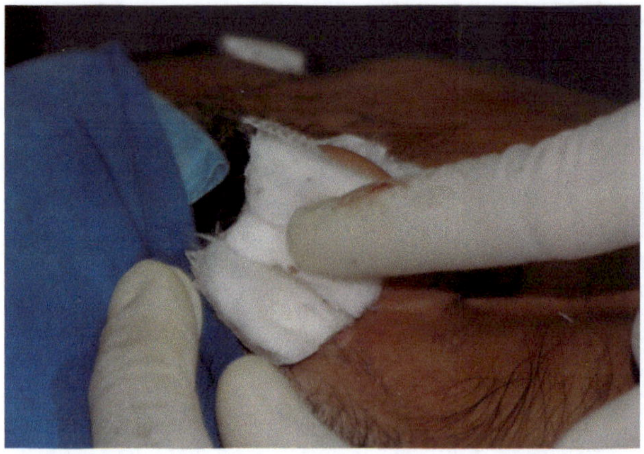

Fig. 18.2.3.12 Dressing with tulle gras and cotton pad

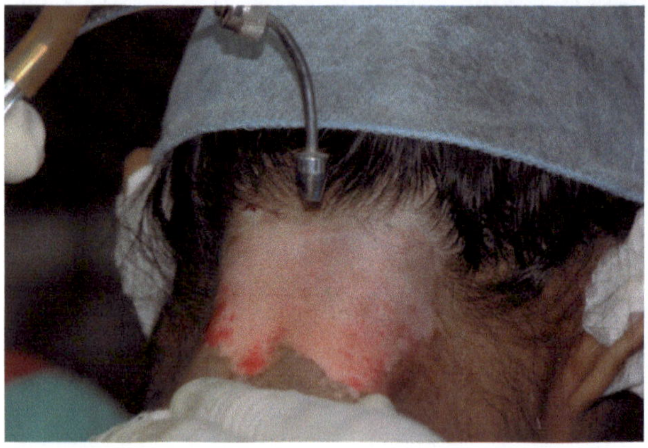

Fig. 18.2.3.13 Microskin grafts sprayed on the dermabraded nape

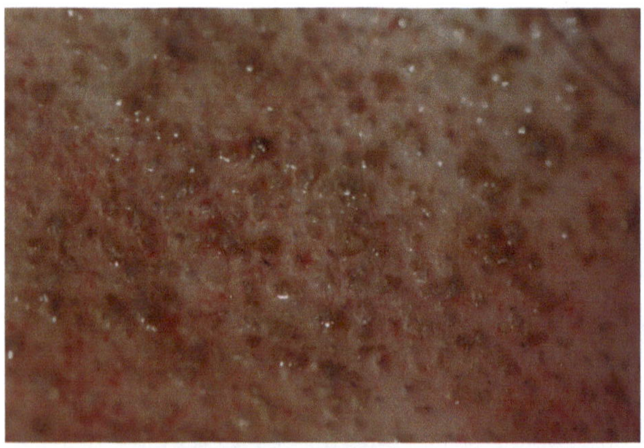

Fig. 18.2.3.14 Close up view of sprayed microskin grafts on the dermabraded nape

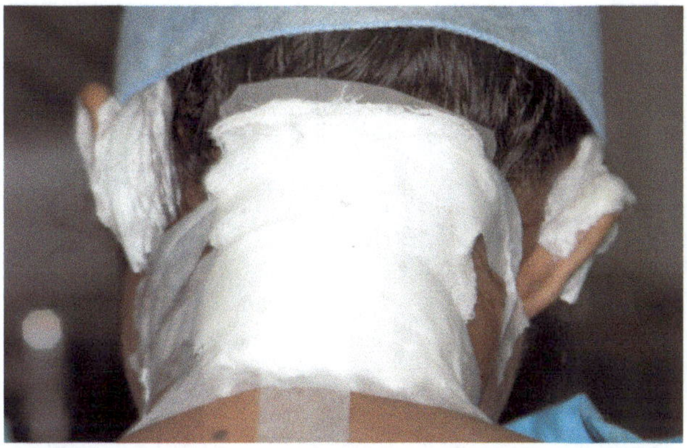

Fig. 18.2.3.15 Nape is dressed with tulle gras and cotton pad. Dressing held in place by hypo allergic paper tape

18.2.4 Post operative results

(Figs. 18.2.4.1-18.2.4.19)

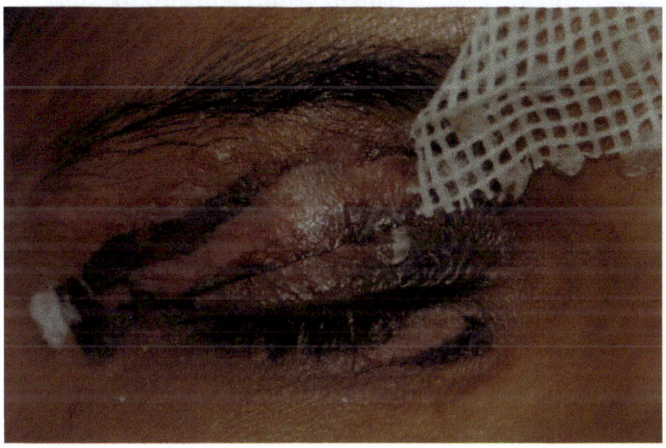

Fig. 18.2.4.1 Ultra thin skin grafting on right upper and lower eyelids on fifth day of bandage removal

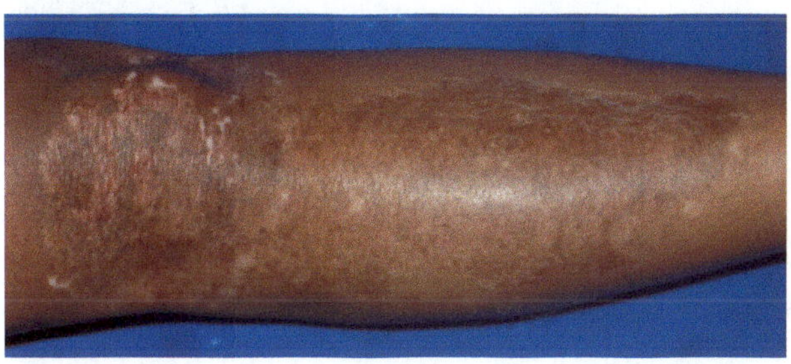

Fig. 18.2.4.2 Near total pigmentation at 5 months on the front of right leg and partial pigmentation in infra-patellar area which was done 3 months back

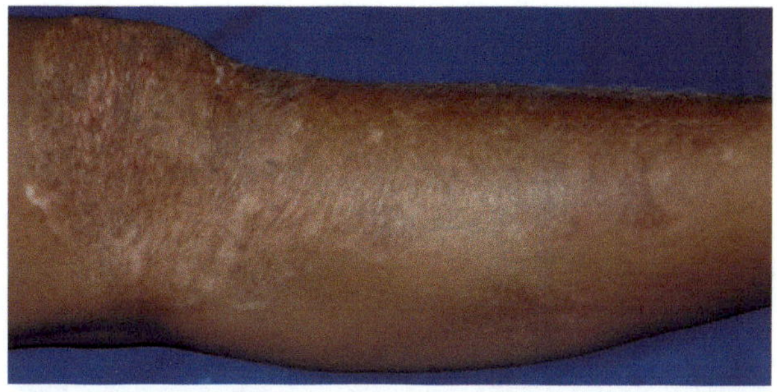

Fig. 18.2.4.3 Near total pigmentation of antero lateral aspect of right leg

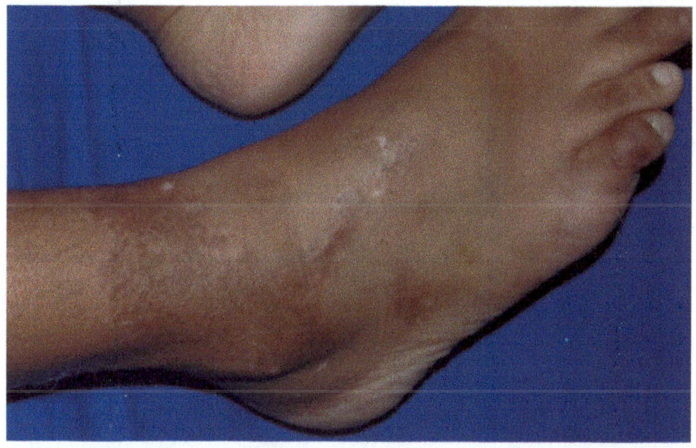

Fig. 18.2.4.4 Repigmentary results at 5 months on the antero-lateral aspect of right ankle

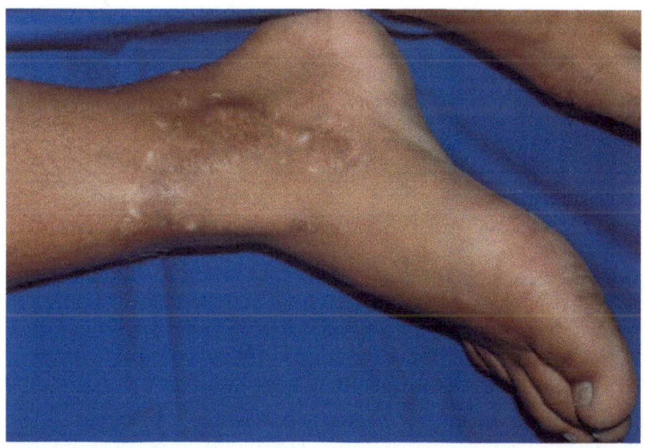

Fig. 18.2.4.5 Repigmentary results at 5 months on the medial aspect of right ankle

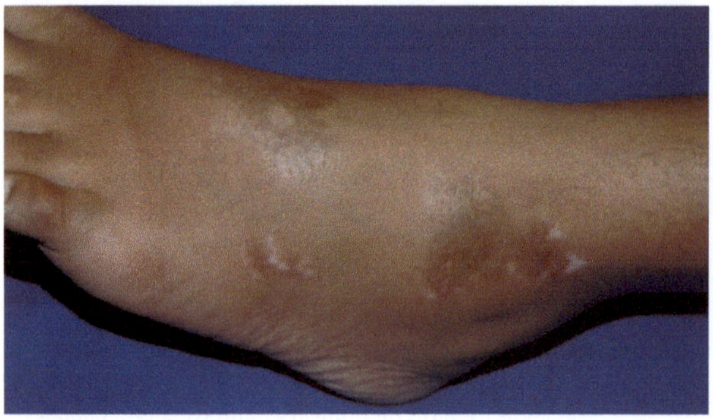

Fig. 18.2.4.6 Repigmentation at 3 months after MSGs on the left foot and the ankle

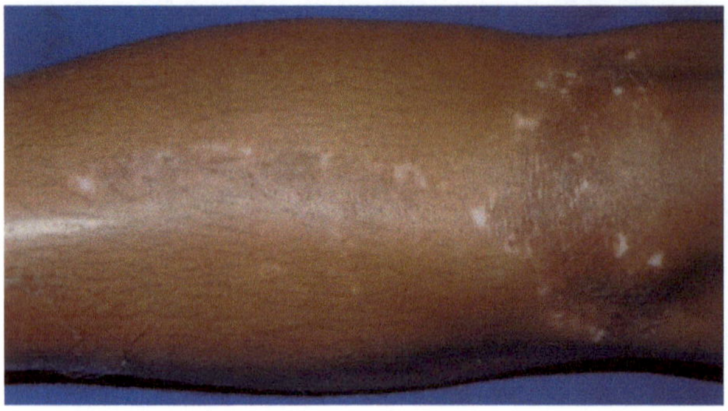

Fig. 18.2.4.7 Repigmentation at 3 months after MSGs on the left knee and front of the leg

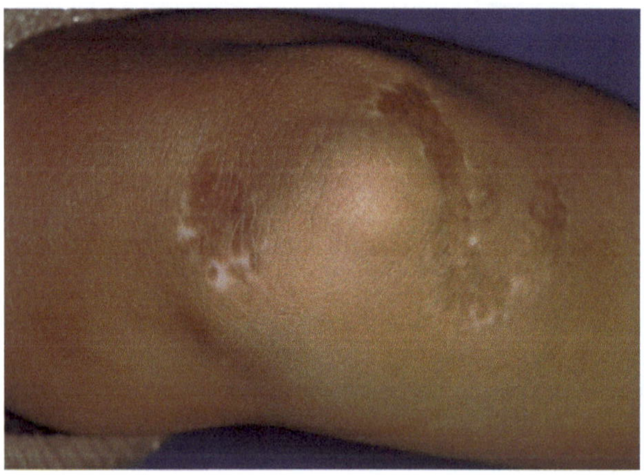

Fig. 18.2.4.8 Repigmentation at 3 months after MSGs on the right elbow

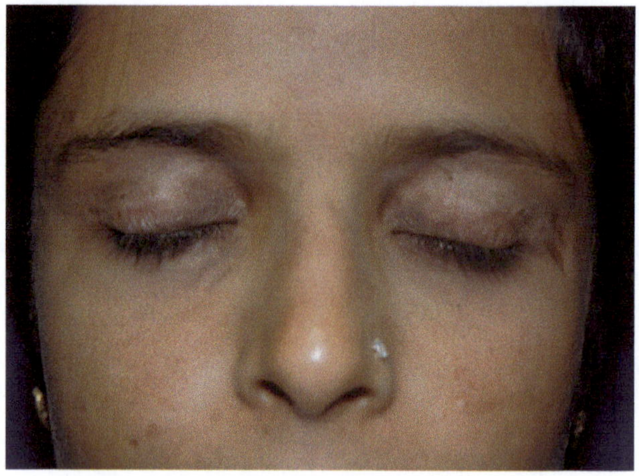

Fig. 18.2.4.9 Repigmentation at 3 months after Ultra thin split thickness skin graft (STSG-UT) on the eyelids

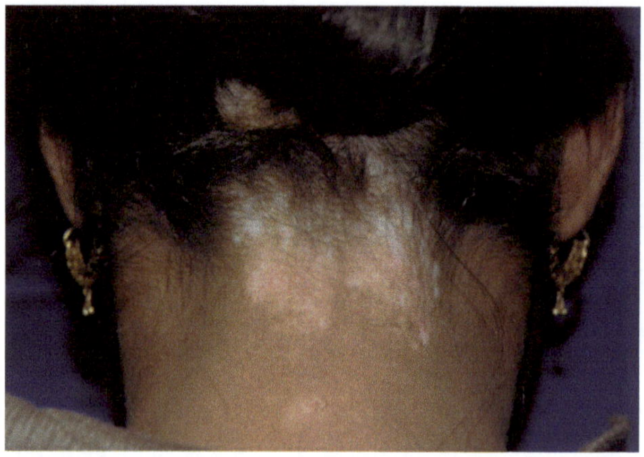

Fig. 18.2.4.10 Repigmentation at 3 months after MSGs on the nape

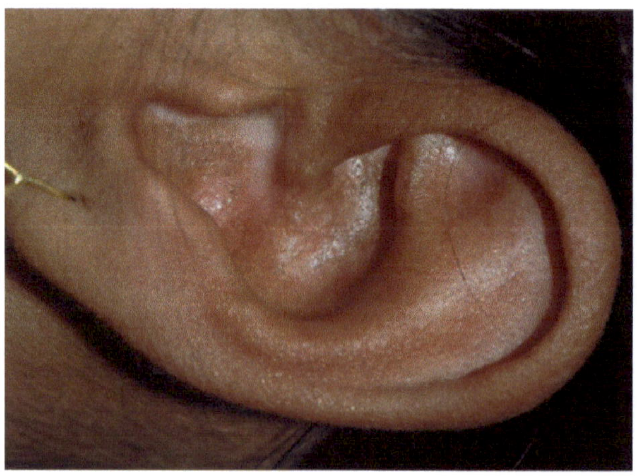

Fig. 18.2.4.11 Repigmentation at 3 months after MSGs on the left pinna

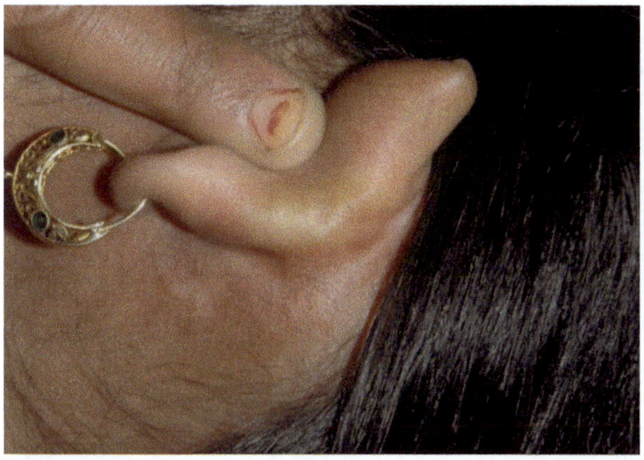

Fig. 18.2.4.12 Repigmentation at 3 months after MSGs on the left post auricular area

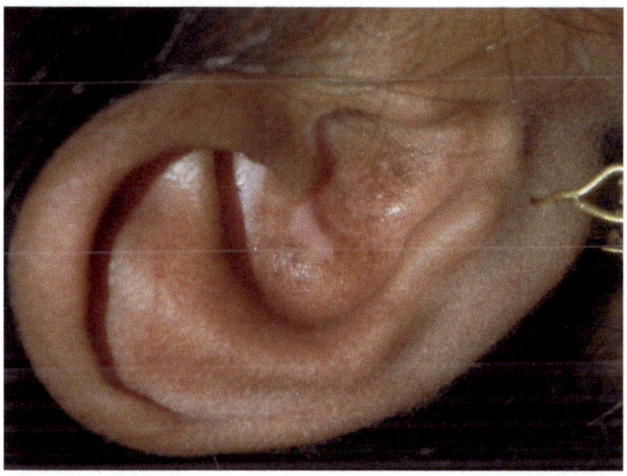

Fig. 18.2.4.13 Repigmentation at 3 months after MSGs on the right pinna

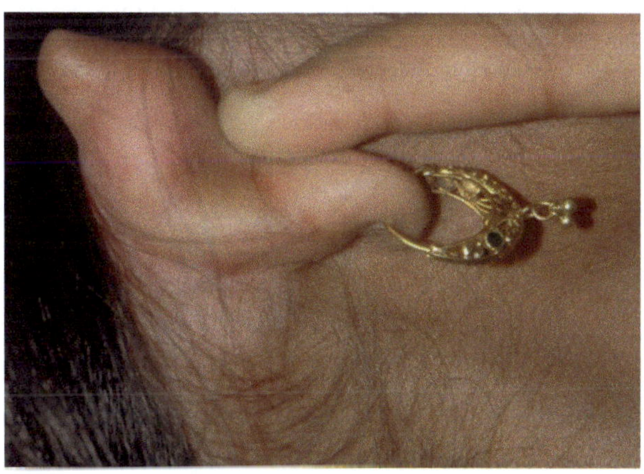

Fig. 18.2.4.14 Repigmentation at 3 months after MSGs on the right post auricular area

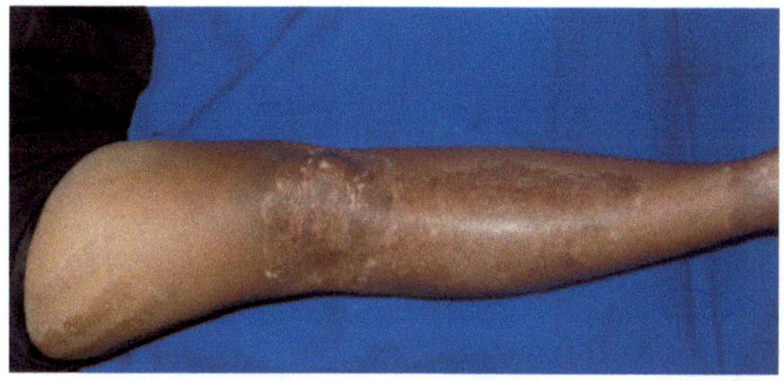

Fig. 18.2.4.15 Fading out donor area defect on the right thigh at 5 months time. Visibility of donor area following graft removal is likely to disappear in a years time

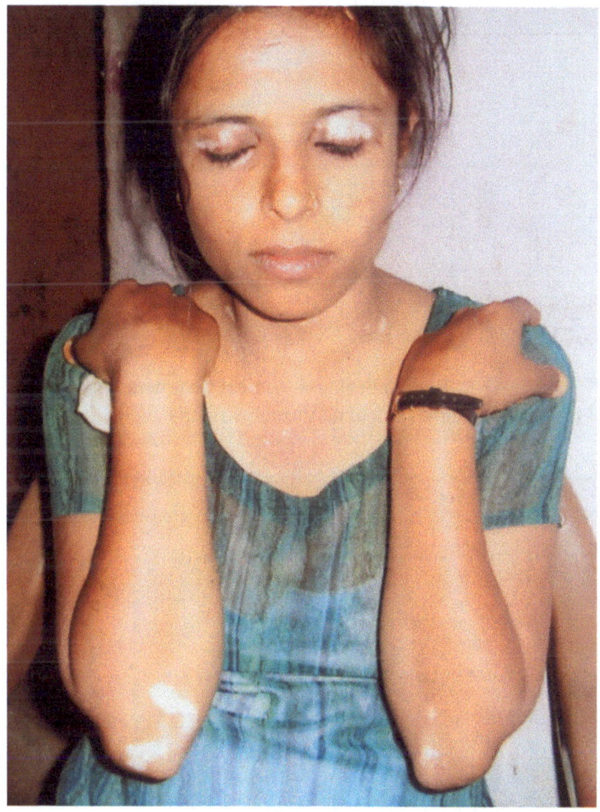

Fig. 18.2.4.16 Pre medical and surgical treatment photograph of patient of Vitiligo vulgaris

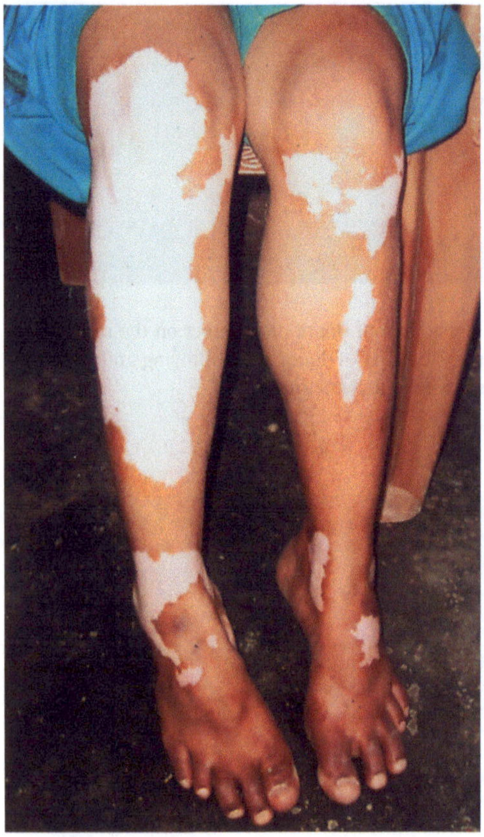

Fig. 18.2.4.17 Pre medical and surgical treatment photograph of both legs of same patient of Vitiligo vulgaris

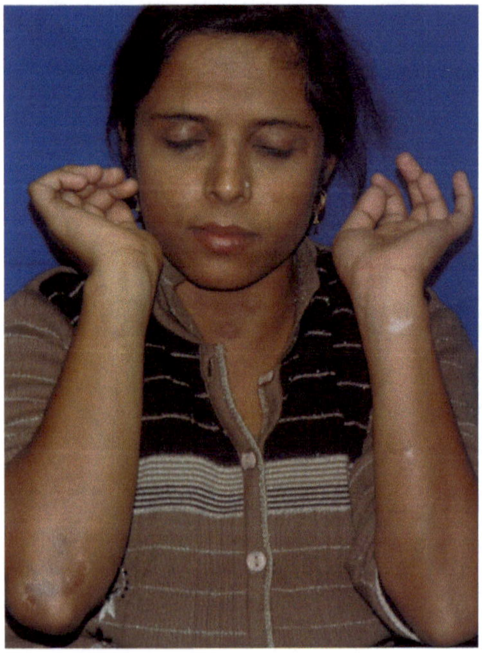

Fig. 18.2.4.18 Post microskin graft results after 3 months. Please note that left wrist area was not Microskin grafted

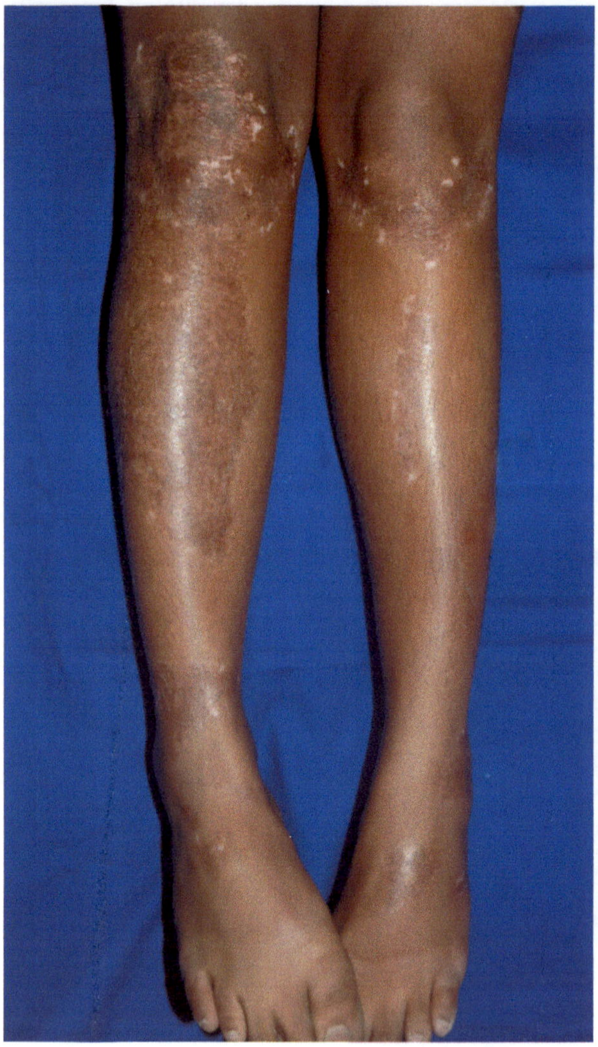

Fig. 18.2.4.19 Post microskin graft pigmentation after 3 months on right infra patellar area and whole of left lower extremity. At 5 months near total pigmentation achieved on right leg and ankle except a small right infra patellar area which was microskin grafted 3 months back

18.3 Case 3 (Extensive Vitiligo)

A 32- year-old male patient of generalized vitiligo controlled medically by steroid and systemic PUVASOL (Psoralen plus ultra violet-A of solar origin). After watching the stability of the disease for 1 year, he was planned for microskin grafting. The patient had white macules over both legs, front of chest, neck, abdomen, flanks, areola, navel and lateral side of hips (Figs. 18.3.1–18.3.23).

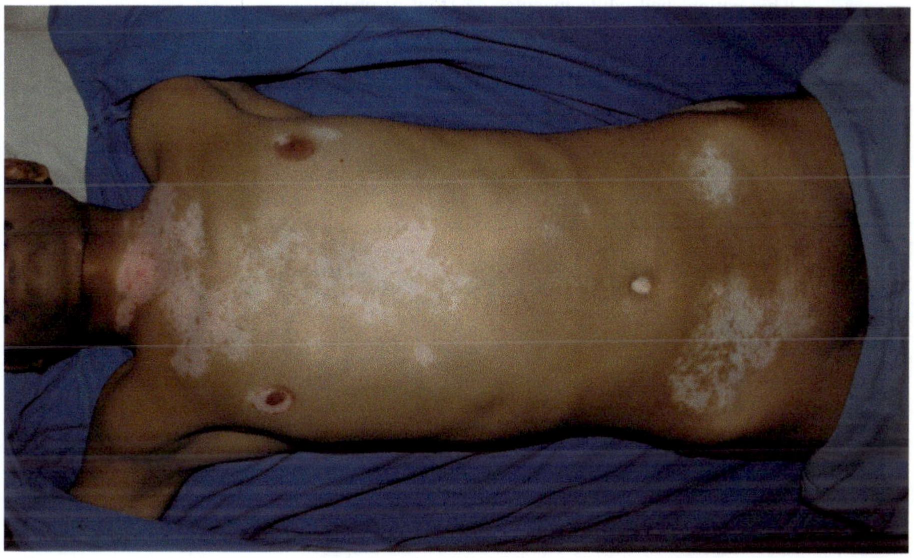

Fig. 18.3.1 This patient had white macules on front of chest, neck, abdomen, flanks, areola, navel and lateral side of hips

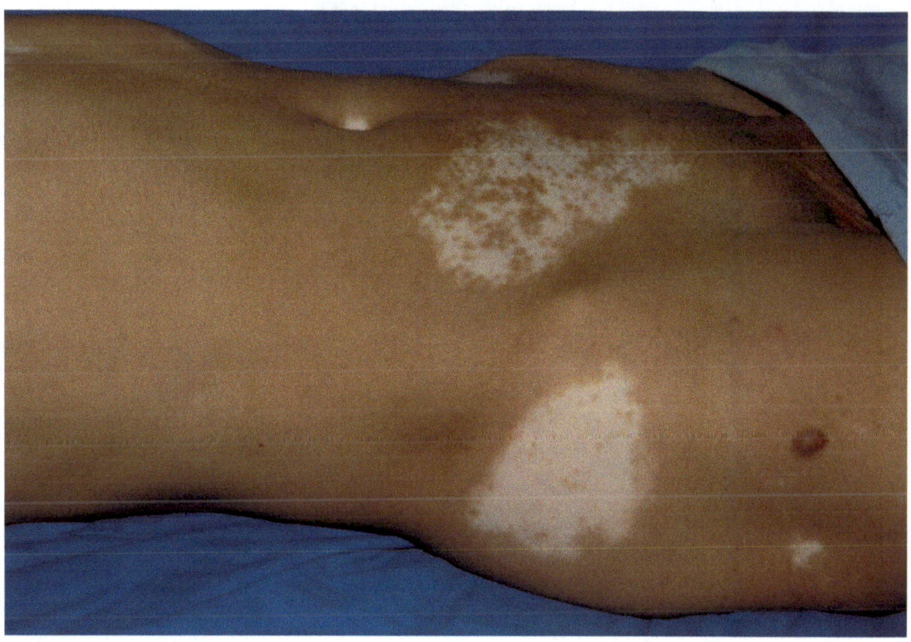

Fig. 18.3.2 This patient had white macules on abdomen, navel and outer side of hip-Close-up view

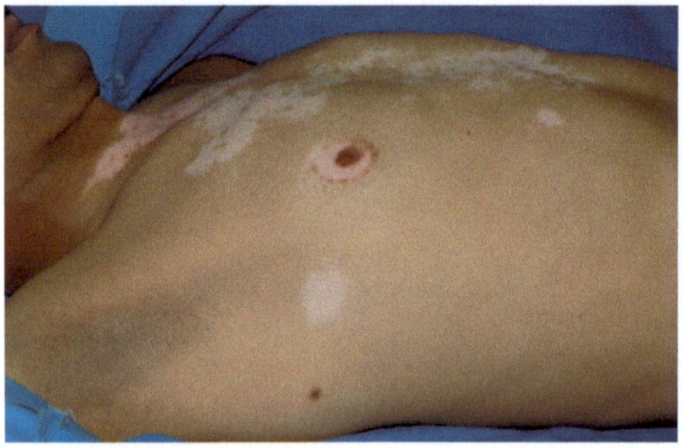

Fig. 18.3.3 This patient had white macules on front of chest, neck, and areola-Right lateral view

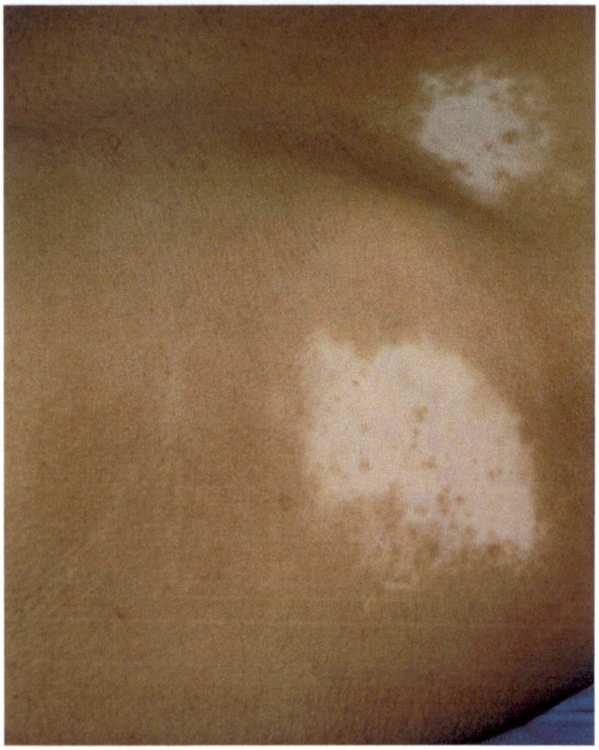

Fig. 18.3.4 This patient had white macules on abdomen, and lateral side of right hip-Close-up view

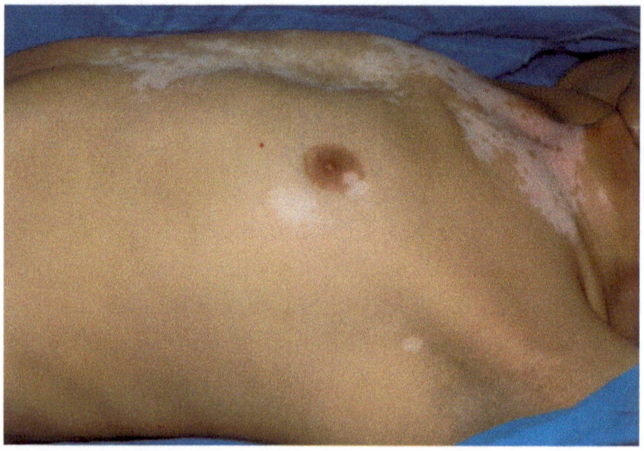

Fig. 18.3.5 This patient had white macules on front of chest, neck, and areola-Left lateral view

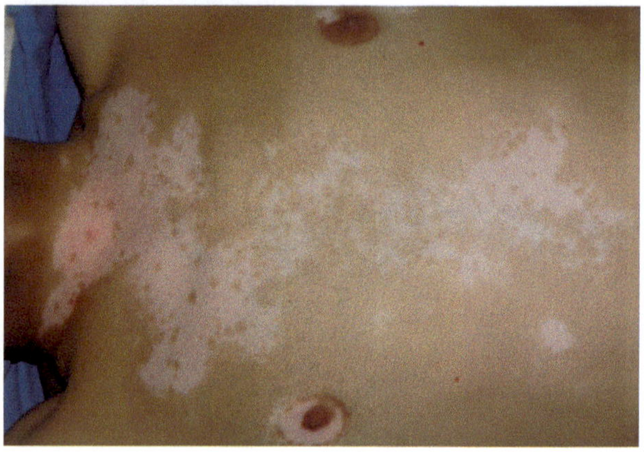

Fig. 18.3.6 This patient had white macules on front of chest, neck, and areola-Close-up view

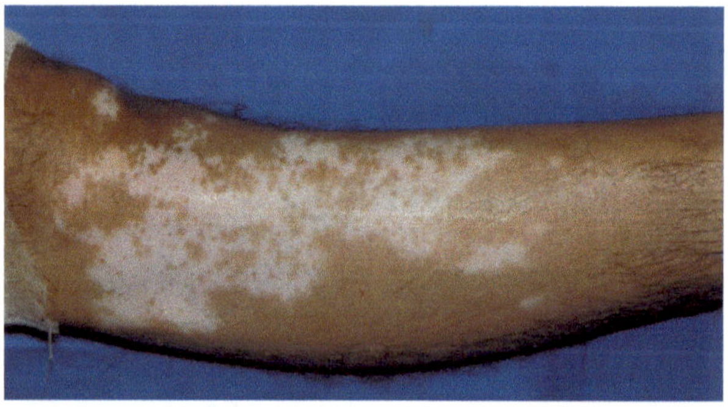

Fig. 18.3.7 This patient had white macules on right leg

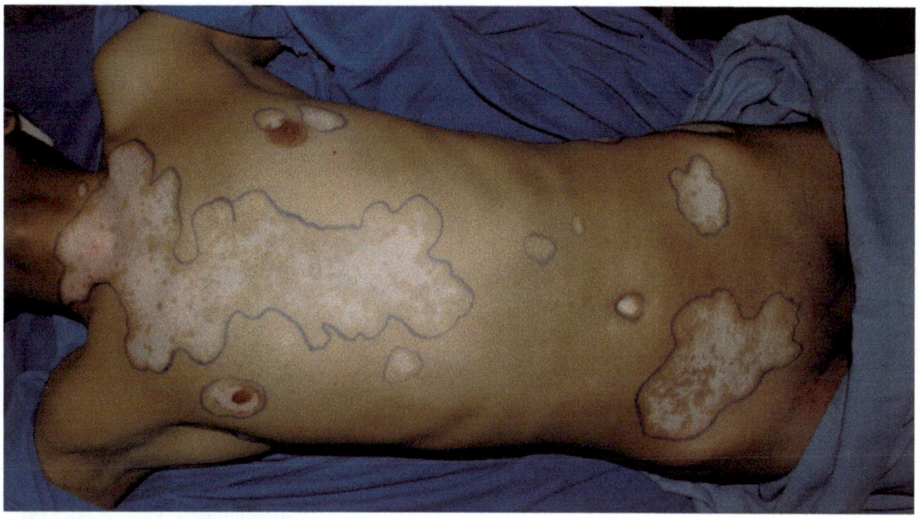

Fig. 18.3.8 Vitiliginous lesions on front of torso marked out with marker

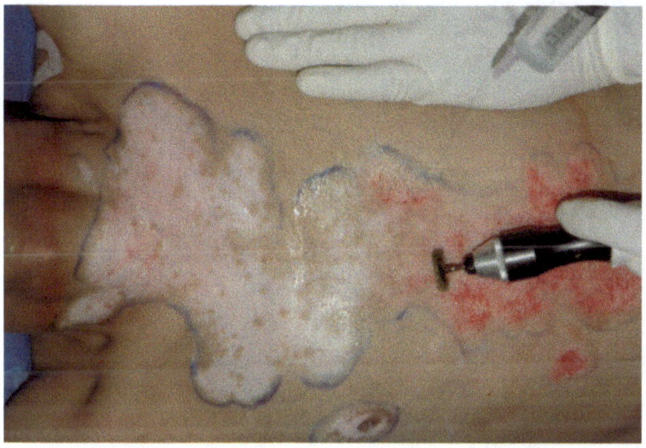

Fig. 18.3.9 Superficial dermabrasion being performed with the help of a rotatory wire brush as shown. Area to be abraded is always kept wet by spraying normal saline with the help of a syringe and a needle. Wire brush is moved perpendicular to the direction of its rotation. Keep moving, otherwise it will produce gouging. Three point retractions are performed by using the surgical assistant's two hands and the surgeon's nondominant hand. Because of the high rate of rotation, the surgical field should be cleared of sponges and towels that may become entangled and injure the physician, the assistant or the patient

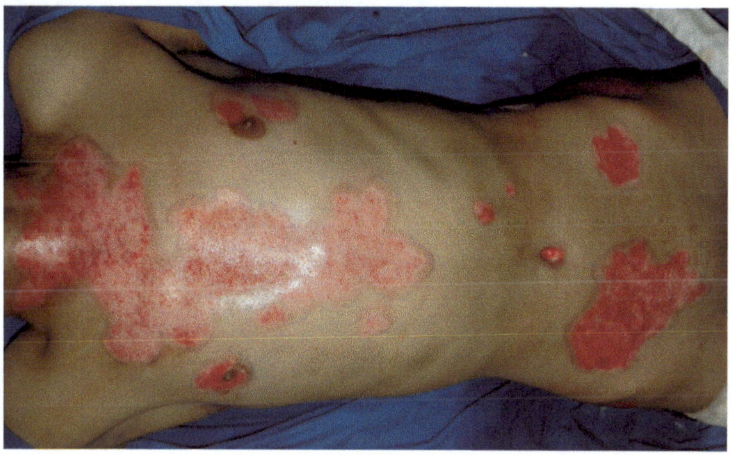

Fig. 18.3.10 Vitiliginous areas on the front of torso after superficial dermabrasion

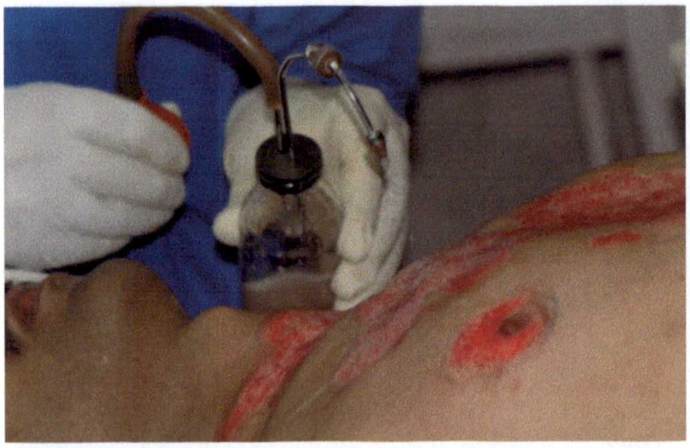

Fig. 18.3.11 Microskin grafts (MSGs) are being sprayed on the dermabraded anterior chest wall. MSGs ejecting out from the nozzle can be seen

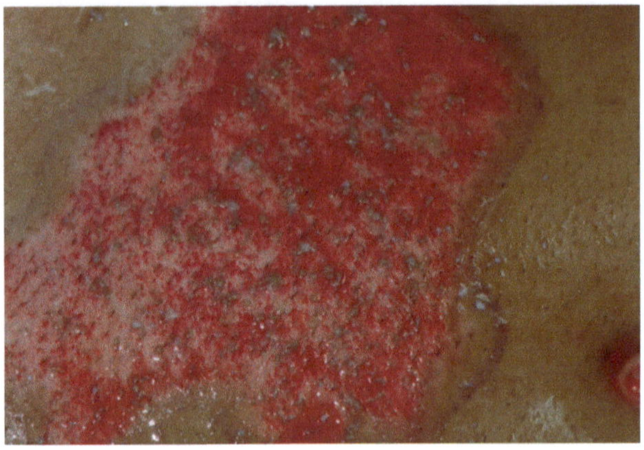

Fig. 18.3.12 Sprayed MSGs lying on the abraded skin surface

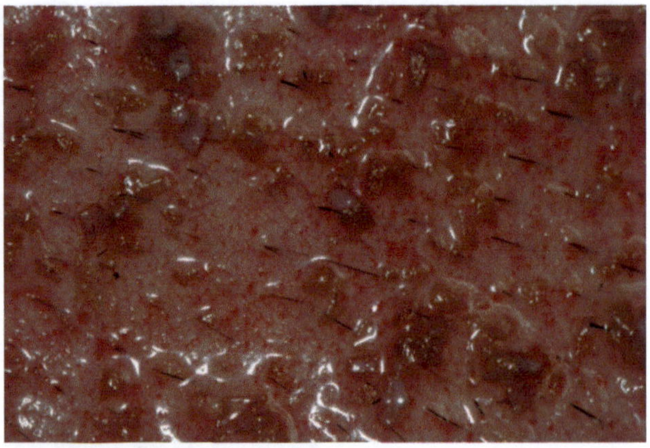

Fig. 18.3.13 Most of the MSGs are lying with the epithelial side up. These particles "take" very well and produces good amount of pigmentation. Few of the MSGs are lying with the epithelial side down. These too "take" by vascularization from the margin. The spread of pigmentation is minimal with the epithelial side down MSGs and most of these grafts bulge out to produce cobblestone effects. In few months these epithelial side down MSGs falls out and the surface becomes smooth without cobblestone effect

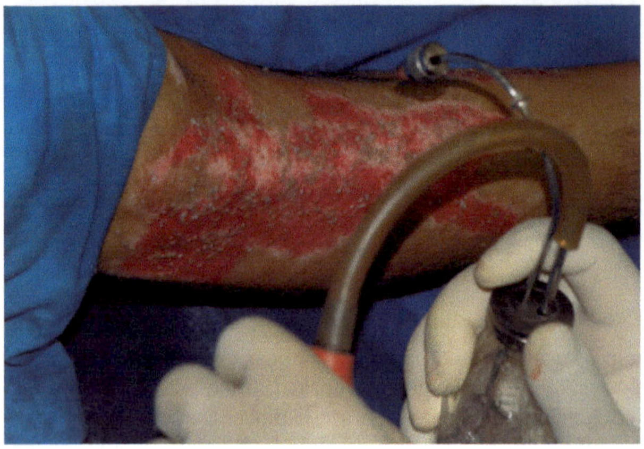

Fig. 18.3.14 Microskin graft sprayed on the dermabraded right leg

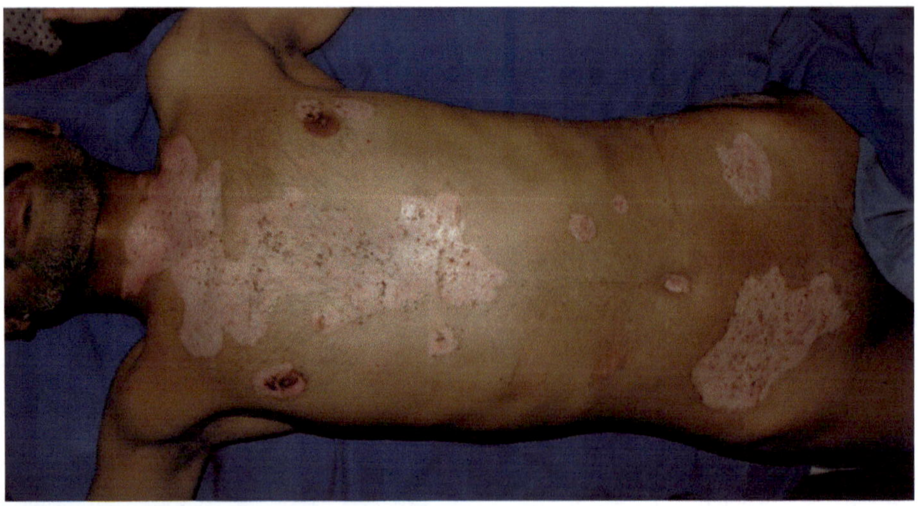

Fig. 18.3.15 Ninth post operative day: all dermabraded and microskin grafted vitiliginous areas on the front of trunk epithelized

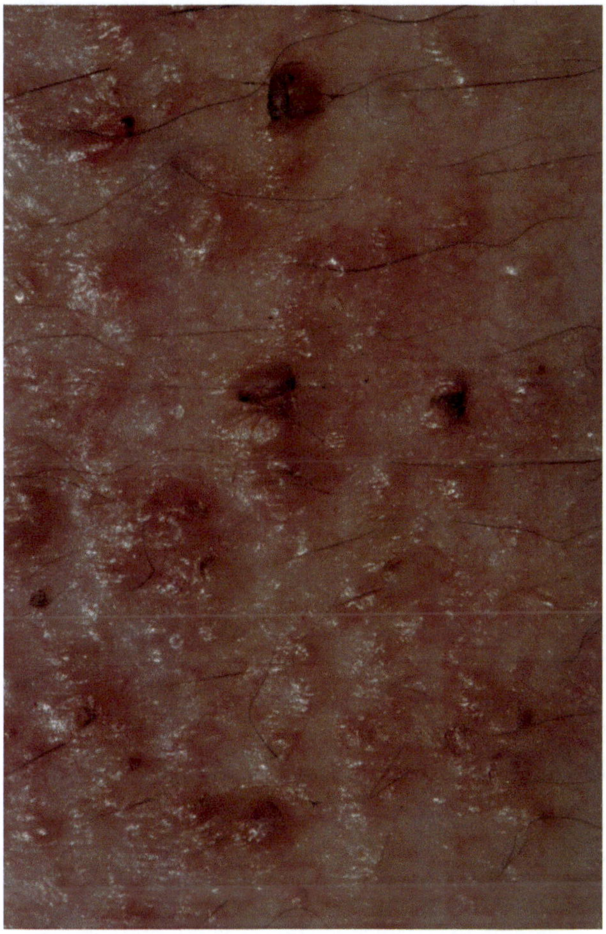

Fig. 18.3.16 Close up view of recipient area. Noticeable evidence of pigmentation even at ninth post-operative day

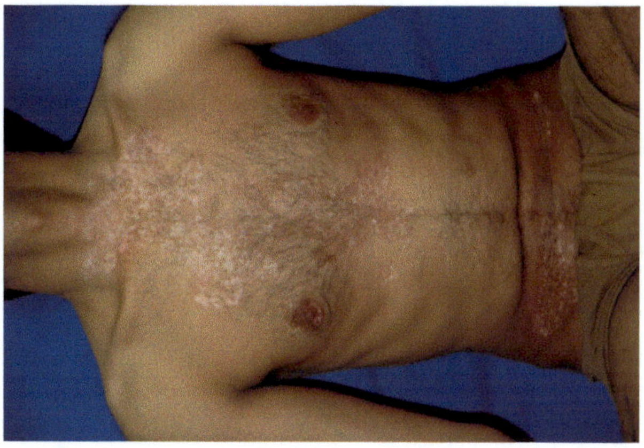

Fig. 18.3.17 Post operative results of repigmentation on front of the chest and the abdomen at 46 days following microskin grafting by spraying method. The amount of pigment spread at this time nearly covered more than 50% of the treated area and expected to complete in 3–4 months time. The PUVASOL (Psoralen plus ultraviolet A of solar origin) therapy continued without interruption and planned to carry upto after complete pigmentation

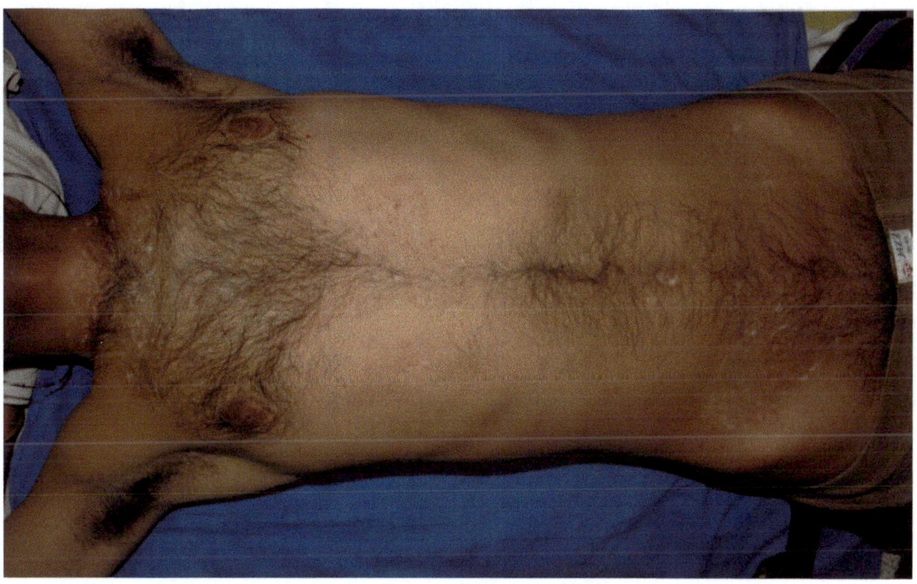

Fig. 18.3.18 Remarkable pigmentation and excellent color match on front of the chest and abdomen at 105th day after microskin grafting done by spraying method. Donor to recipient area expansion ratio was used 1:10–1:15

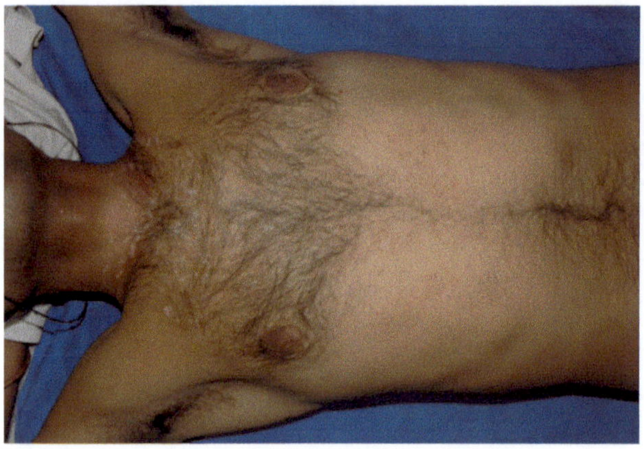

Fig. 18.3.19 Front of the chest. Remarkable pigmentation and excellent color match on front of the chest at 105th day after microskin grafting done by spraying method

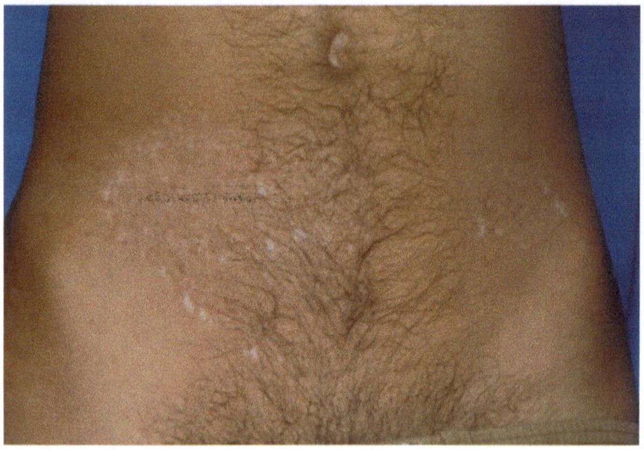

Fig. 18.3.20 Remarkable pigmentation and excellent color match on abdomen at 105th day after microskin grafting done by spraying method

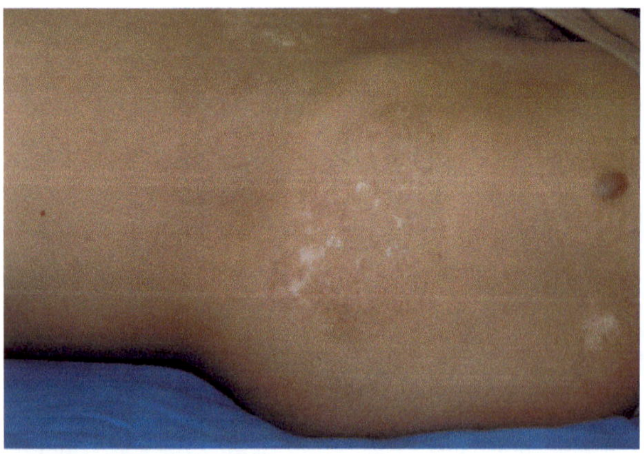

Fig. 18.3.21 Lateral side of the right hip. Remarkable pigmentation and excellent color match at 105th day after microskin grafting done by spraying method

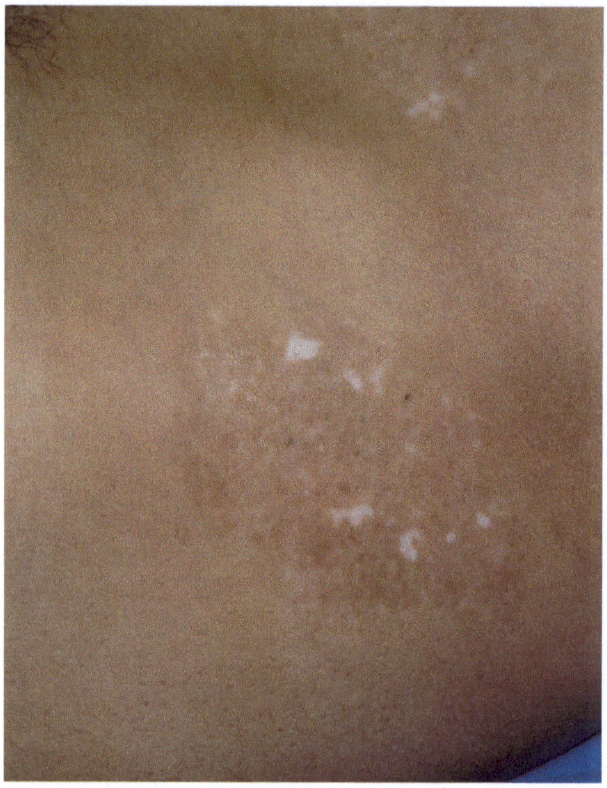

Fig. 18.3.22 Lateral side of left hip. Remarkable pigmentation and excellent color match at 105th day after microskin grafting done by spraying method

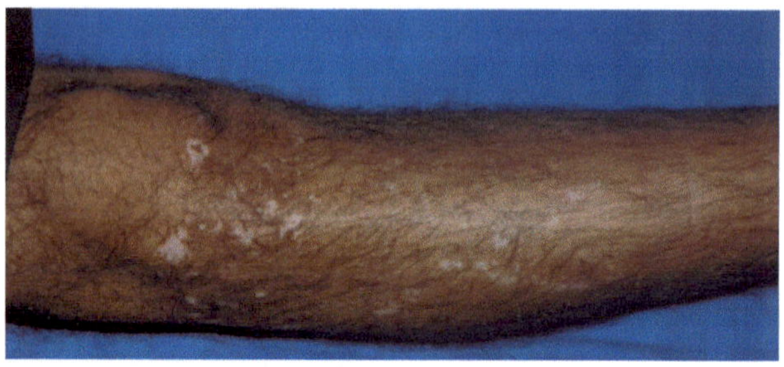

Fig. 18.3.23 Anterior aspect of the right leg. Remarkable pigmentation and excellent color match at 105th day after microskin grafting done by spraying method. Pigmentation would likely to improve in coming months of time

18.4 Case 4 (Vitiligo of Lip and Eyelids)

A 21- year-old female having vitiligo for 11 years duration on her lip and eyelids. Vitiligo is stable for more than a year (Figs. 18.4.1–18.4.10).

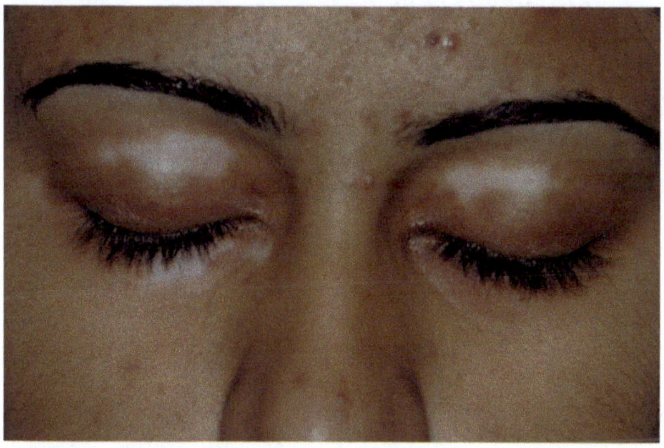

Fig. 18.4.1 Vitiligo on eyelids

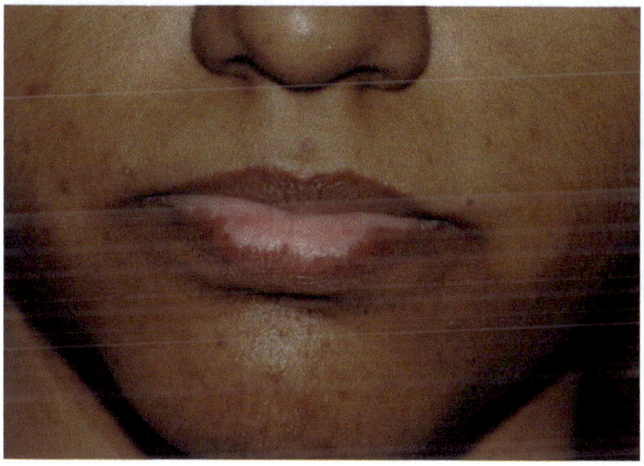

Fig. 18.4.2 Vitiligo on lip

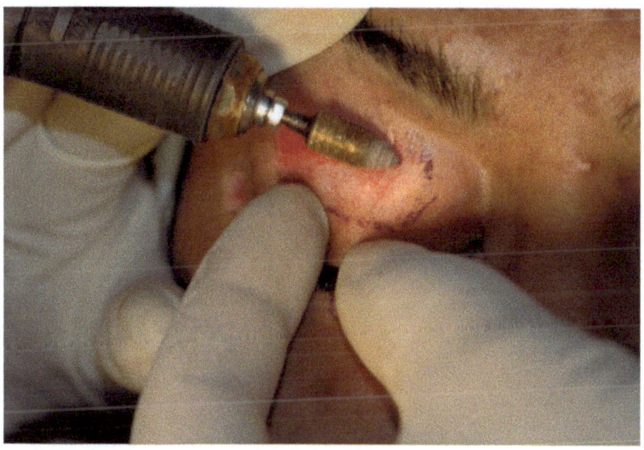

Fig. 18.4.3 Very gentle superficial dermabrasion is done with the help of diamond fraise on her eyelids

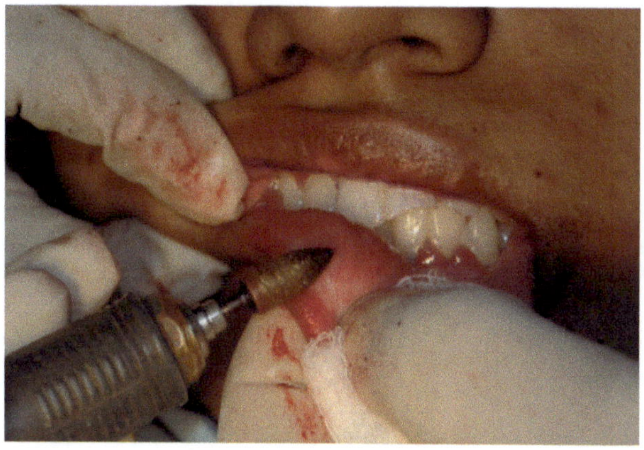

Fig. 18.4.4 Dermabrasion of the lower lip

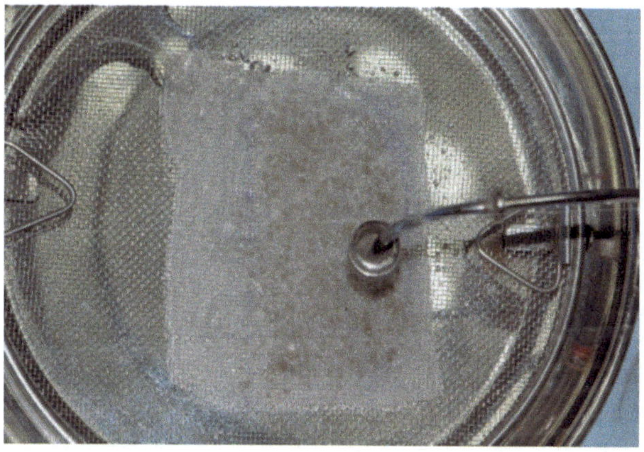

Fig. 18.4.5 Microskin grafts are sprayed on the muslin sheet as shown by the spraying device

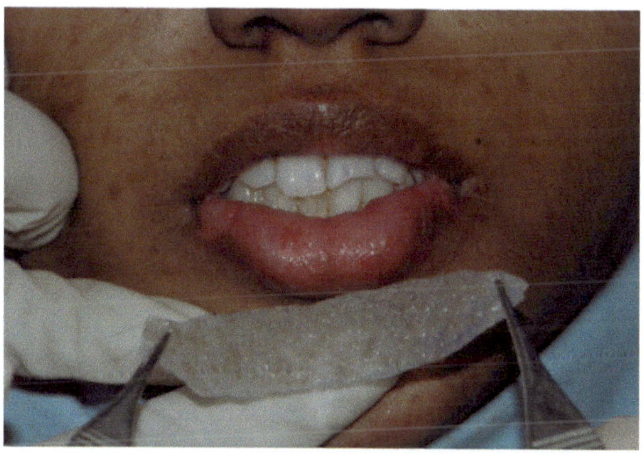

Fig. 18.4.6 Muslin sheet carring MSGs, cut according to the size of the vitiliginous dermabraded area and being applied on the lower lip. Microskin grafts on the surface of muslin sheet are very well seen

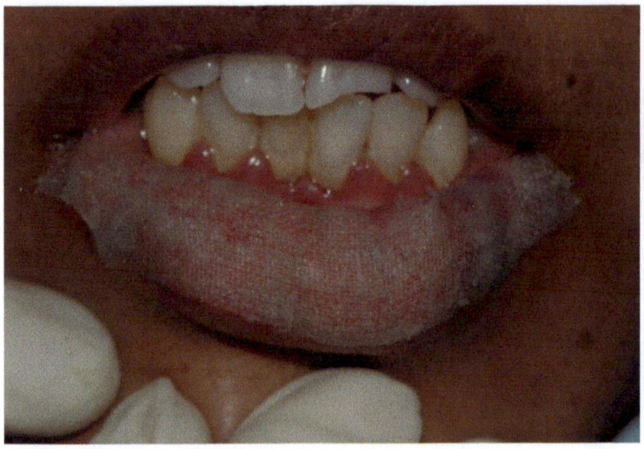

Fig. 18.4.7 Muslin sheet stuck to the lip as such or may some times need a few fine sutures to fix at periphery

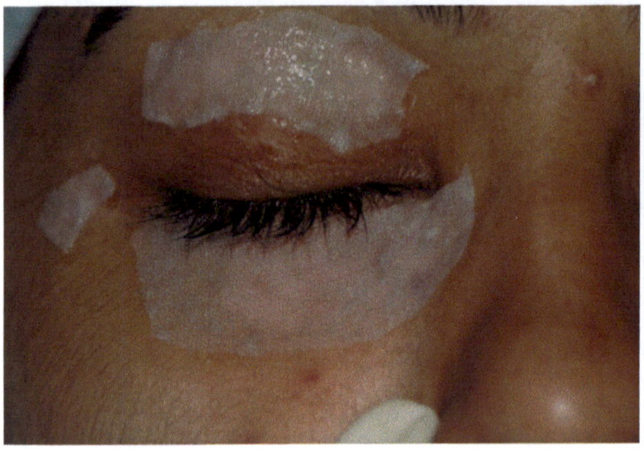

Fig. 18.4.8 MSGs carrying muslin sheet cut pieces are applied over dermabraded eyelids and fixed carefully. Eyelids may be padded for 3–5 days to avoid the movement of the microskin grafts

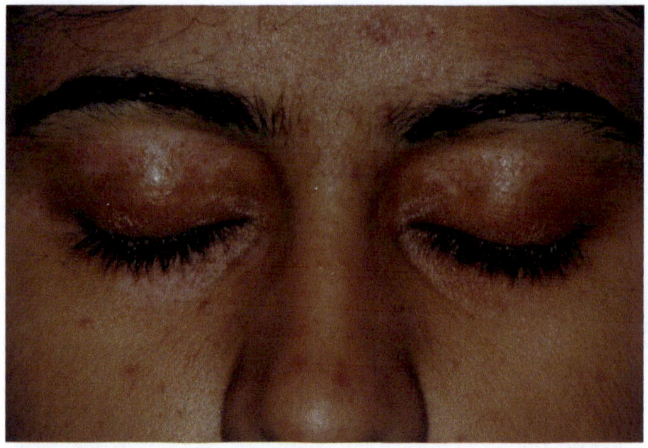

Fig. 18.4.9 Remarkable repigmentation at 20th post operative day of the eyelids

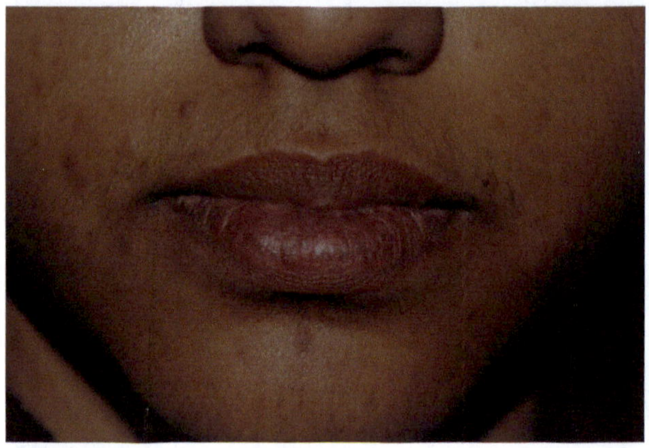

Fig. 18.4.10 Remarkable repigmentation at 20th post-operative day on the lower lip

18.5 Case 5 (Vitiligo of Lip-Tip Syndrome)

This young girl had vitiligo of lips and tip of fingers. Such cases are most of the time refractoy to medical treatments. In this patient only lower lip was dermabraded and Microskin grafted. (Figs. 18.5.1 and 18.5.2).

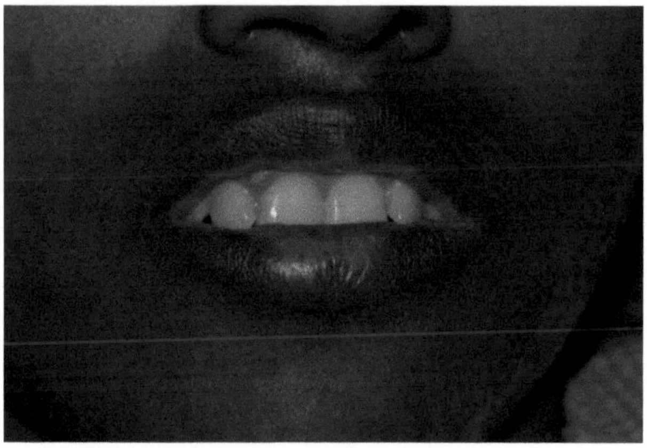

Fig. 18.5.1 Lip-tip syndrome:vitiligo lower lip

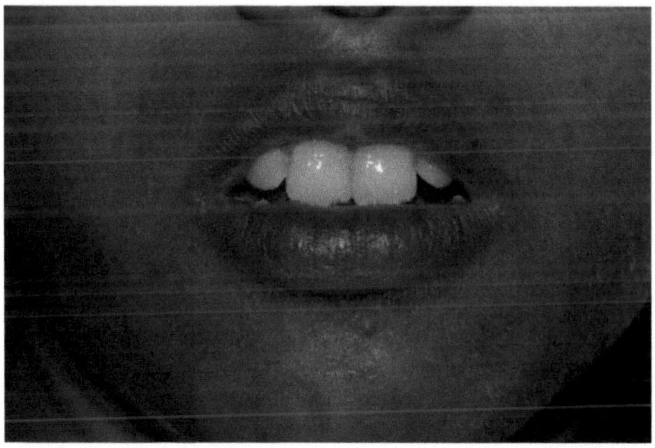

Fig. 18.5.2 Pigmentation achieved at 5 months on the lower lip after Microskin grafting

Part IV

Surgical Outcomes

19 Complications Involved in Various Surgical Techniques

Postoperative complications, such as peripheral hypopigmentation, delayed hyperpigmentation, milia, inclusion cysts, achromic fissures, thick margins, stuck-on appearance, are quite common with split thickness skin grafts (STSG). In the recipient site, cobblestone appearance was the predominant complication in punch grafts, whereas, hyperpigmentation and thickening of grafts were common in suction blister epidermal grafts (STSG-BE). The color match was statistically significant in punch grafts, when compared to STSG-BE. Time taken for satisfactory color match with thin split-thickness skin graft is about 4–9 months. Punch grafts give a better color match than STSG-BE. Slight hyperpigmentation is common, especially when ultra thin split thickness graft (STSG-UT) has been used. No scars or indurations were seen in the donor areas in case of ultra thin split thickness graft.

19.1 Recipient Area Complications (Figs. 19.1–19.12)

- Hyperpigmentation
- Hypopigmented borders
- Cobblestoning
- Contact dermatitis to topical medication
- Inclusion cysts
- Thick margins/stuck-on appearance
- Variegated appearance
- Infection
- Scarring

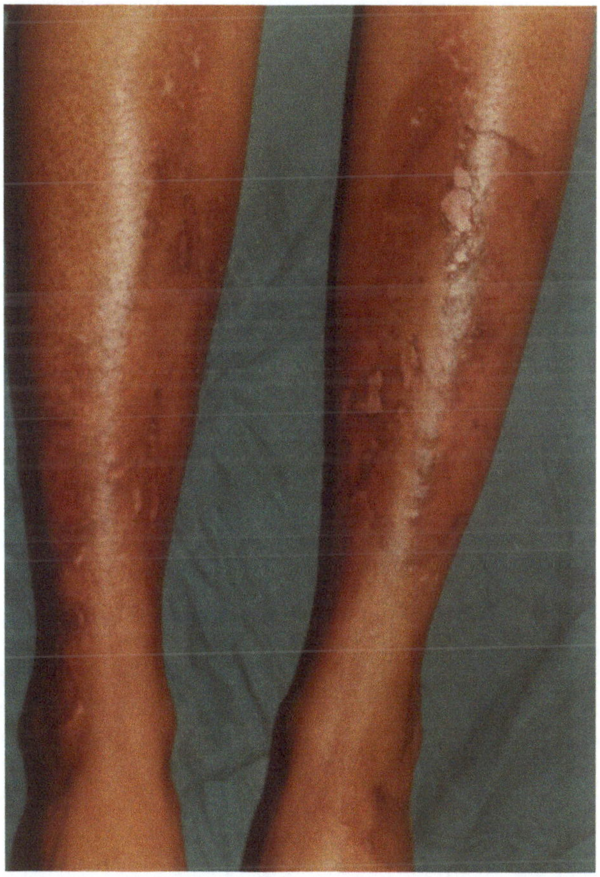

Fig. 19.1 Achromic fissures at the recipient area following thin split thickness skin graft with good color match

D. K. Gupta, *Microskin Grafting for Vitiligo*,
DOI: 10.1007/978-1-84882-605-2_19, © Springer Science + Business Media B.V. 2009

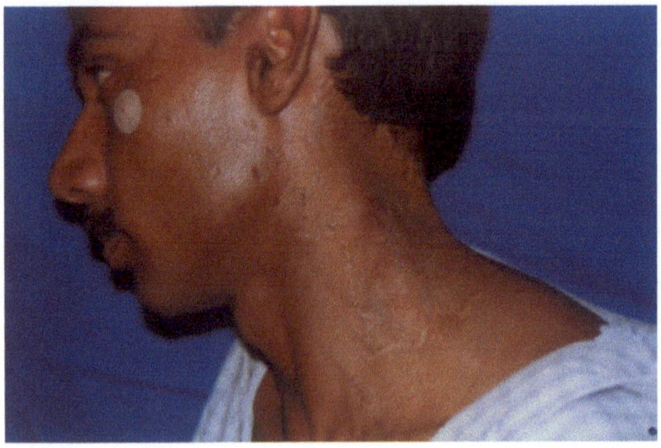

Fig. 19.2 Hypopigmented borders at the recipient area following thin split thickness (STSG-T) skin graft with good color match

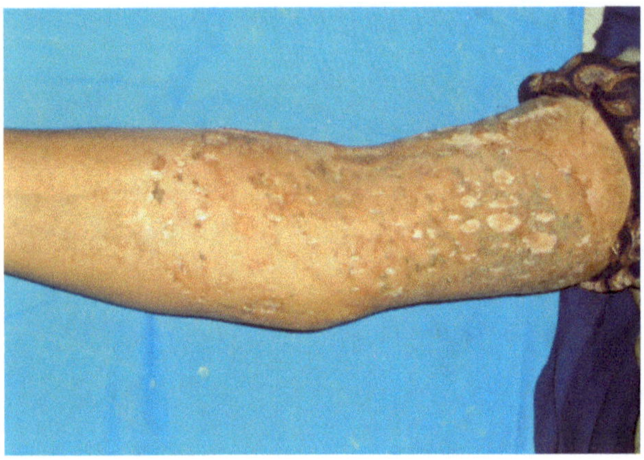

Fig. 19.3 Thick margins, achromic fissures and stuck-on appearance at the recipient site following medium thickness skin graft (STSG-M)

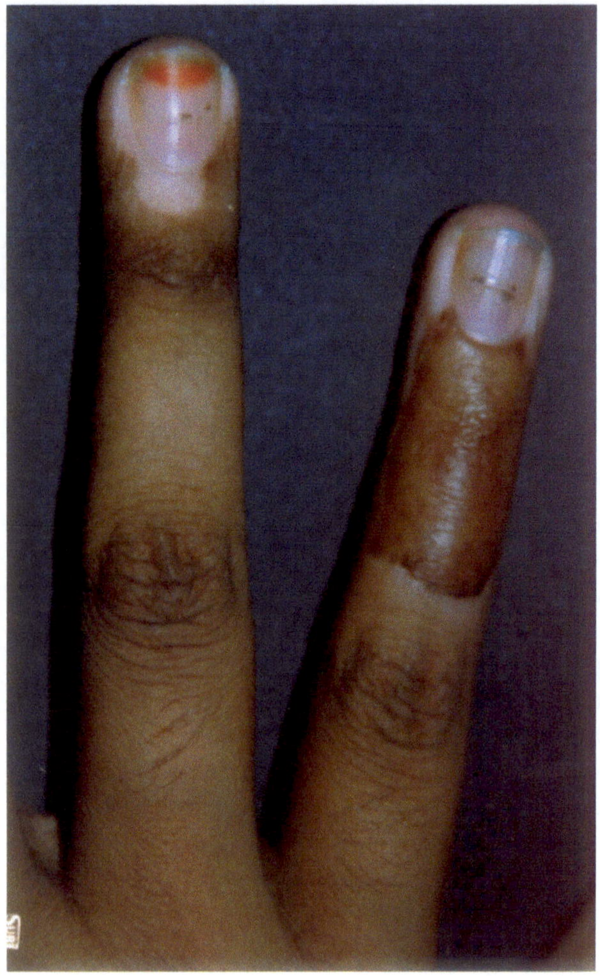

Fig. 19.4 Stuck-on appearance at the recipient site of the right ring finger following thin spilt thickness skin graft

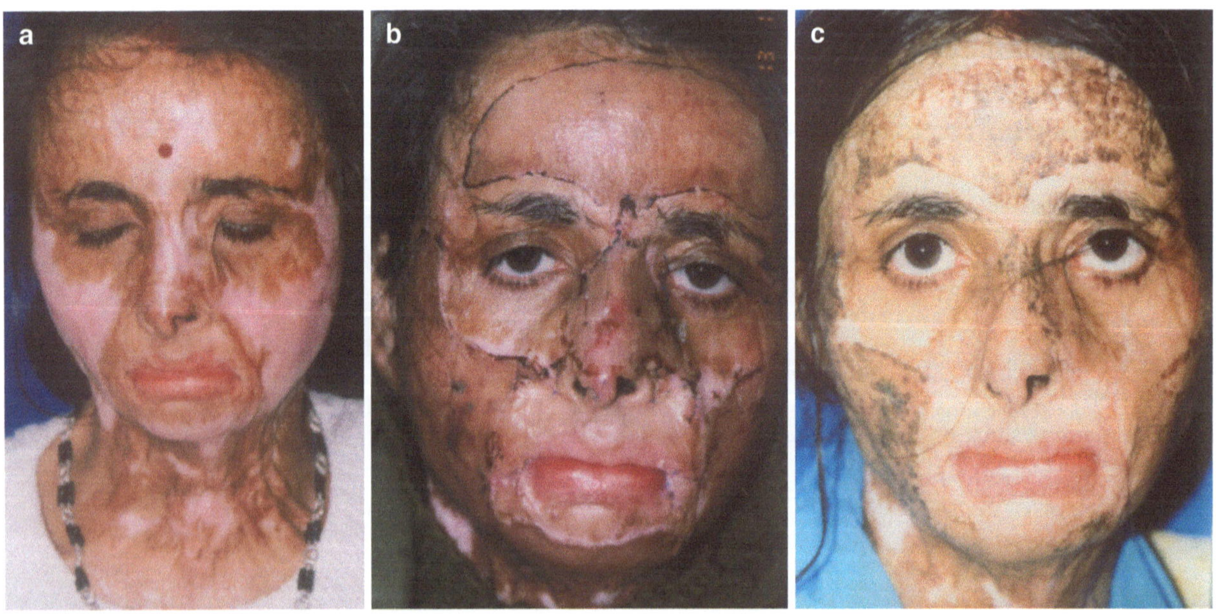

Fig. 19.5 (**a–c**) Inclusion cysts and variegated appearance following thin split thickness skin graft (STSG-T) on the face for post burn leukoderma

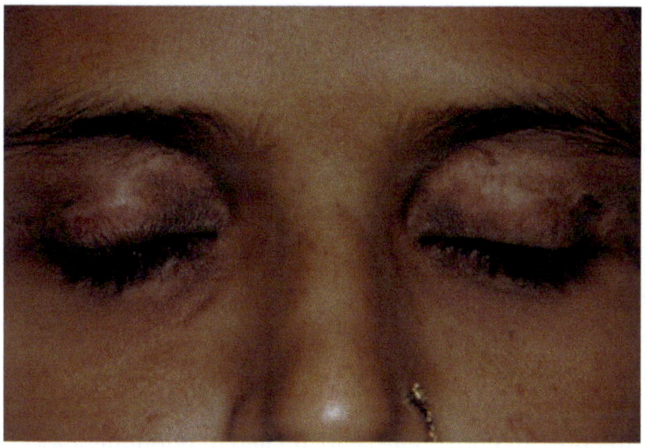

Fig. 19.6 Shrivelled and fragmented ultra thin graft used for eyelid vitiligo. Cosmetic results improved with time

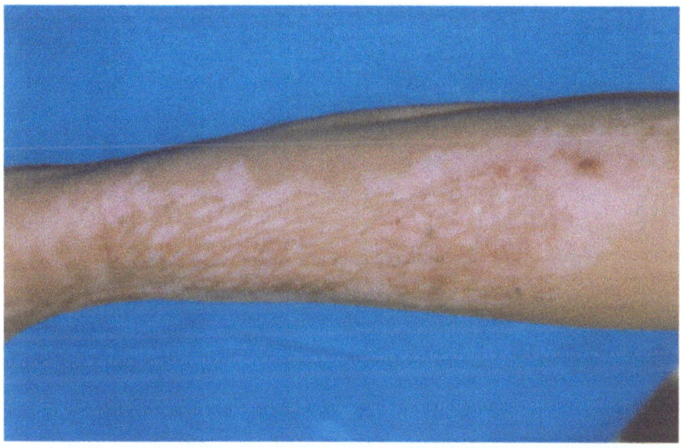

Fig. 19.7 Cosmetically unacceptable mesh pattern on the leg following expanded mesh grafting

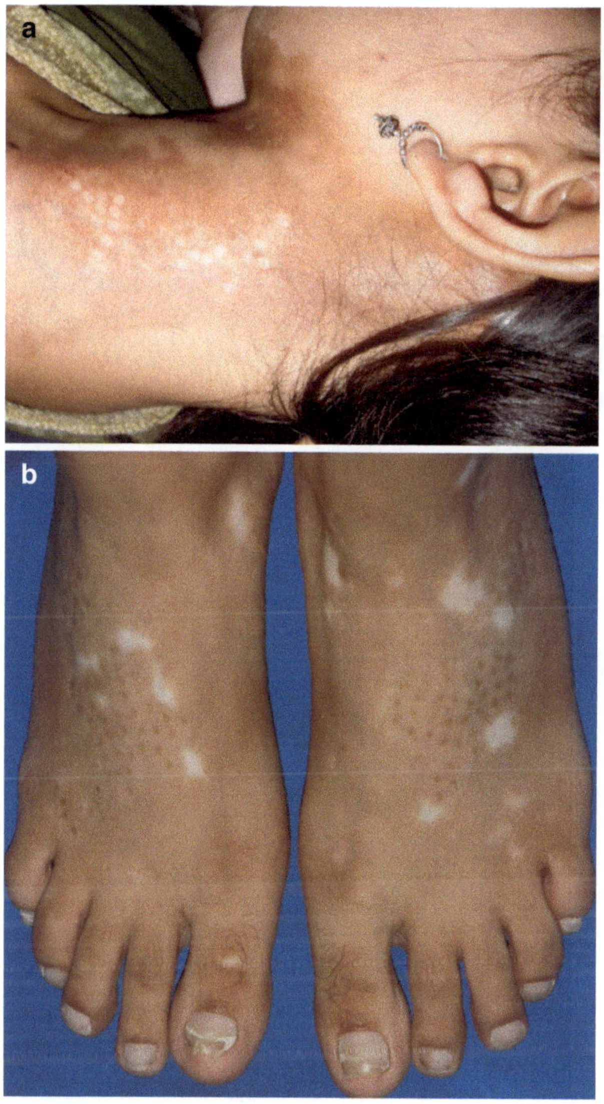

Fig. 19.8 (**a**, **b**) Variegated appearance following punch grafting with partial depigmentation of the punch grafts

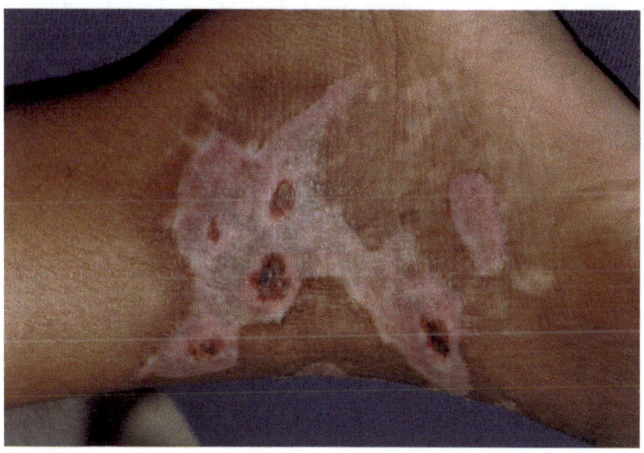

Fig. 19.9 Focal infection at the recipient site with scab formation

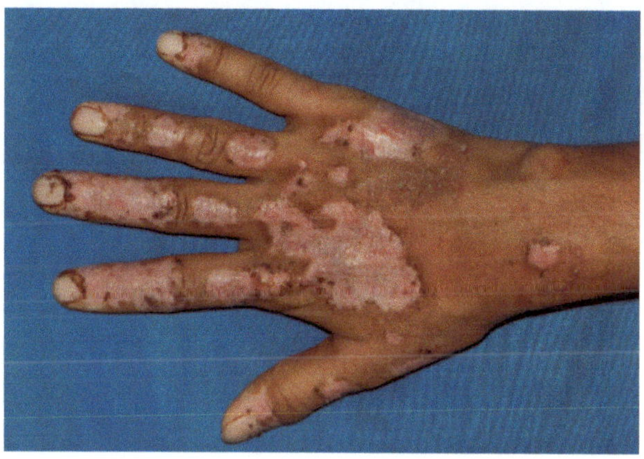

Fig. 19.10 Contact dermatitis following the use of vaseline tulle gras on the ulnar side of the dorsum of hand

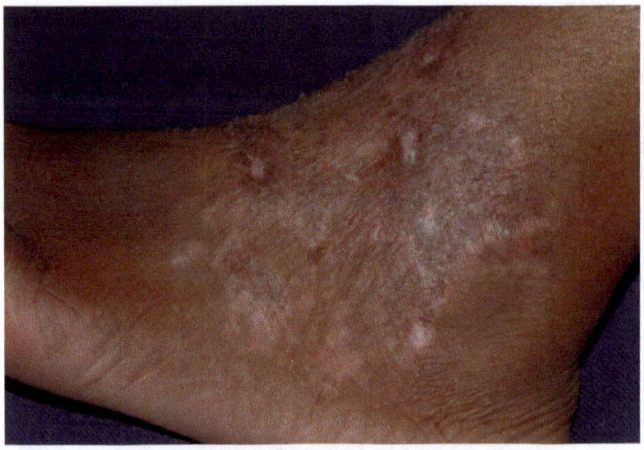

Fig. 19.11 Dermatitis at the recipient site controlled by steroid cream

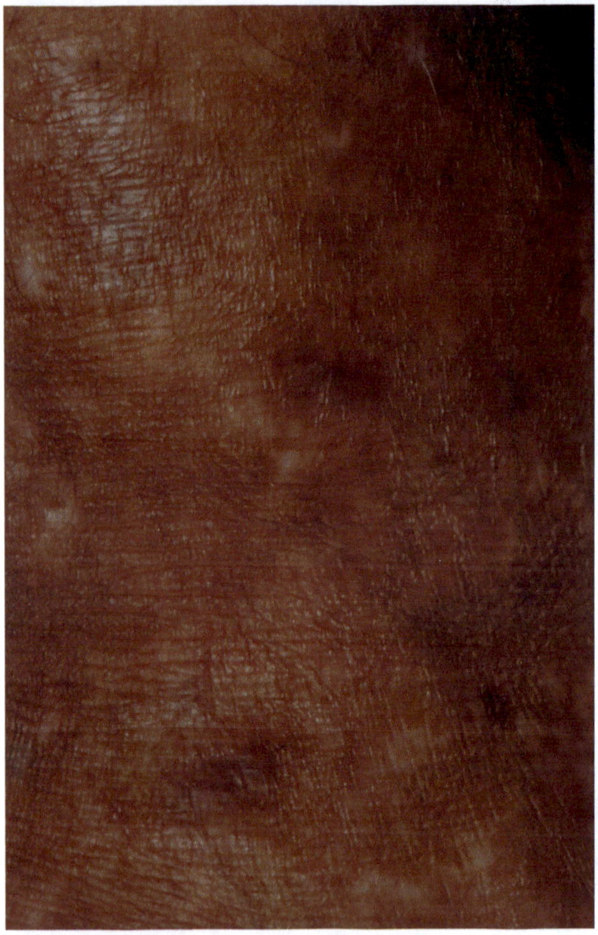

Fig. 19.12 Hyperpigmented suction blister grafts

In the donor site, superficial scarring and hypopigmentation are the common findings in Punch grafts, whereas, hyperpigmentation is the main problem in STSG-BE and STSG-UT.

There is a minimal risk of scarring at the donor site, if very thin or ultra thin grafts are taken. The irregularity of pigmentation, which is noticed following all surgical procedures, is likely to improve in due course. Depigmentation developed at the donor site in patients with progressive generalized unstable vitiligo. Infection, hypertrophic scarring and hypopigmentation are common when you remove thicker grafts from donor areas.

19.2 Donor Area Complications (Figs. 19.13–19.19)

- Hyperpigmentation
- Hypopigmentation
- Scarring
- Koebner phenomenon
- Infection

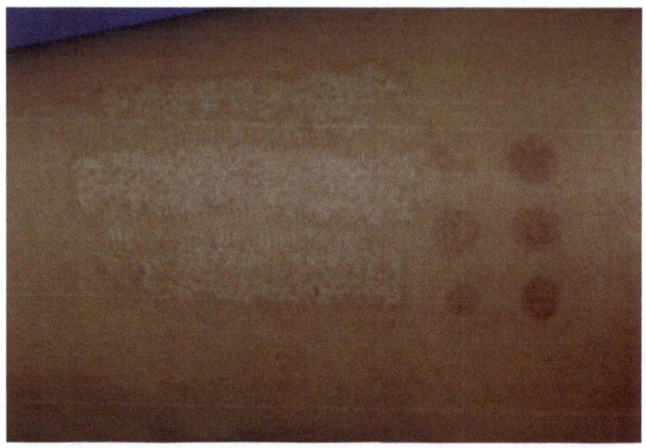

Fig. 19.13 Hyperpigmentation following blister graft removal and hypopigmentation after thin split thickness skin graft harvesting from the thigh

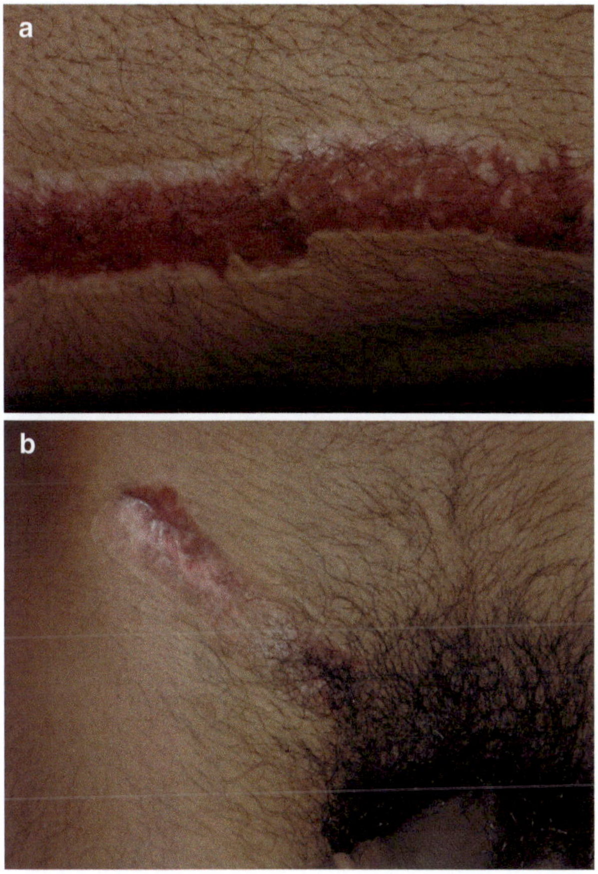

Fig. 19.14 (**a**, **b**) Hypertrophic scar formation after thick split thickness skin graft cutting from the thigh and the groin

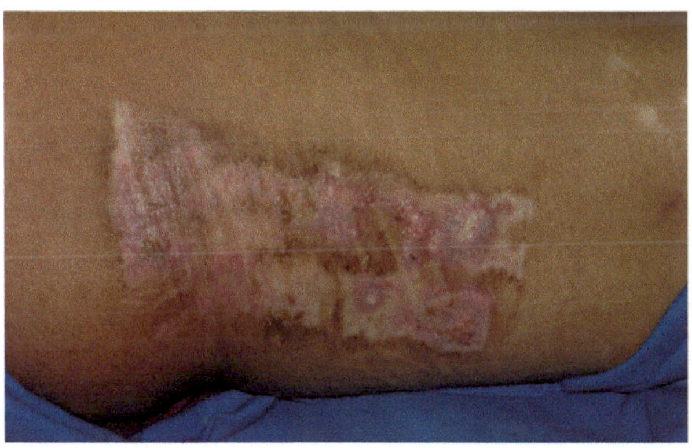

Fig. 19.15 Donor area infection managed by frequent washing and dressing

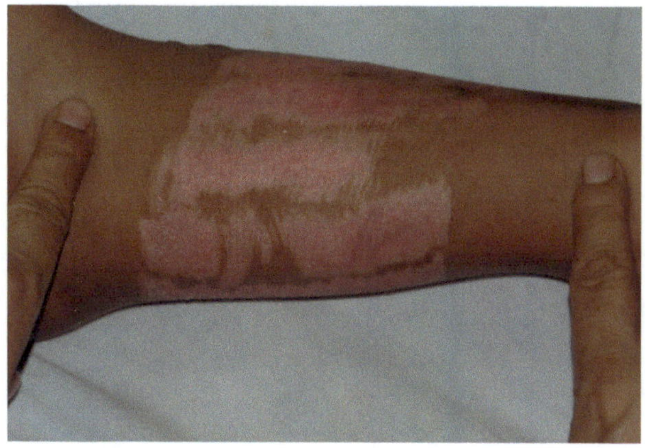

Fig. 19.16 Ideally donor area should heal within 11–13 days following very thin or ultra thin graft cutting. Initially healed hypopigmented area becomes hyperpigmented followed by normal color match in about 4–9 months time

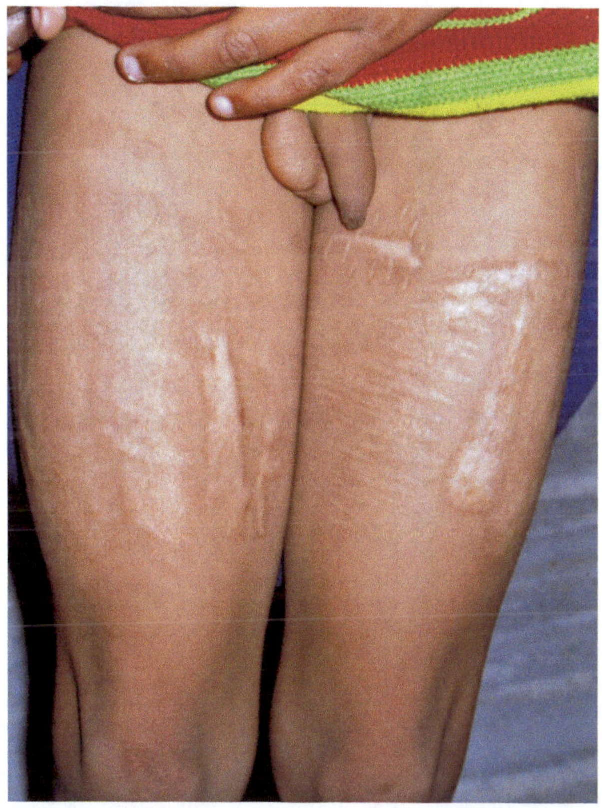

Fig. 19.17 Multiple donor area deformity due to graft cutting by a novice surgeon

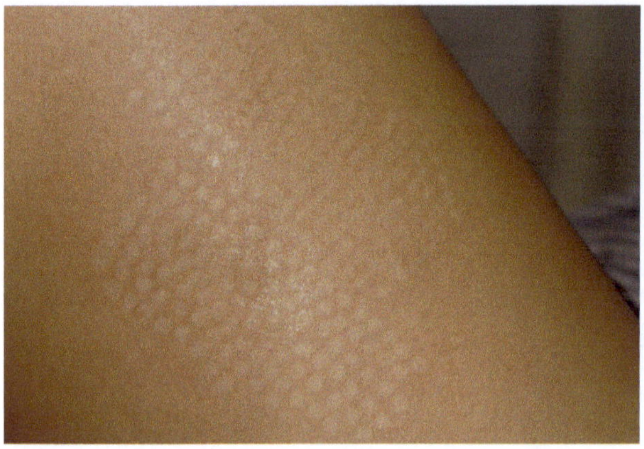

Fig. 19.18 Donor area scarring after punch graft cutting from the thigh

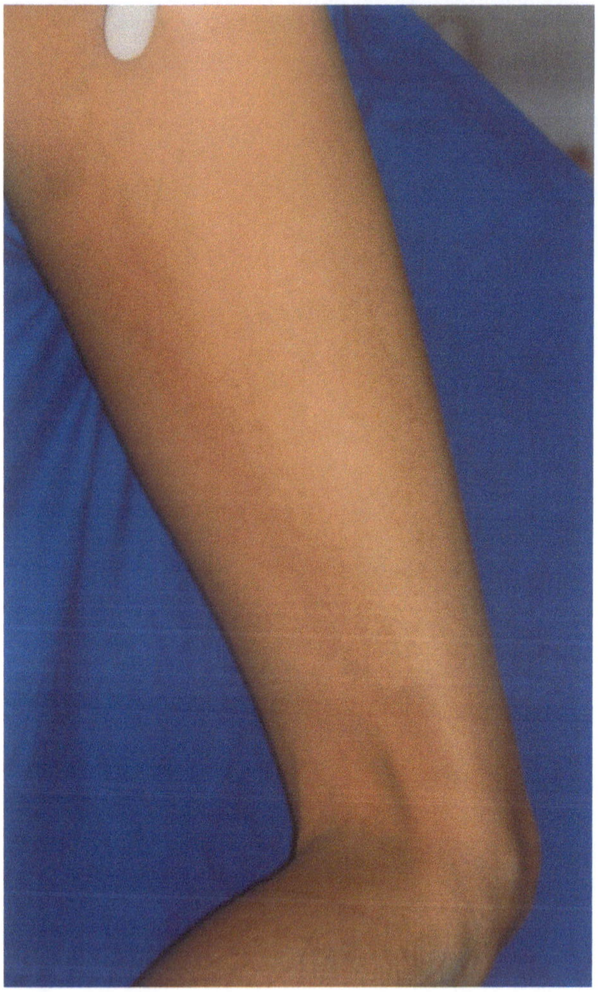

Fig. 19.19 Hardly visible donor area defect after a big sheet of thin graft harvested from the thigh at 1 year

Outcome of Various Techniques of Vitiligo Surgery

20

Vitiligo surgeries are not without complications. Most authors have claimed good-to-excellent results (60–95% repigmentation) with the surgical method that they had adopted depending upon the type, size, site and stability of vitiligo lesions, age and color complexion of the patient, and whether local or systemic PUVA/PUVASOL was used post-operatively.[1–17]

Overall, better results are reported in focal and segmental vitiligo (75–95%) than in generalized vitiligo. Younger (20–30 years) and darker complexioned patients have better results. Comparatively, acral areas, malleoli, knees, and elbows are less responsive to surgery. Smaller patches respond better. Addition of PUVA/PUVASOL therapy enhances repigmentation and increases the success rate (90–95%).

On an average, STSG-UT, STSG-T and STSG-BE, yield 1:1 coverage of the affected area. In MPG, the perigraft spread of pigment is 4–15–folds. However, the limitation of MPG is that cosmetic acceptability is not very good. Noncultured epidermal cell suspension gives a coverage of 3–10 times the biopsy specimen size, but requires tedious perioperative steps. The best expansion obtained is with pure cultures (mixed or pure melanocytes). But, facilities for culture are expensive, available at few centers, and need technical support.

The overall success rate of transplantation procedures for generalized and segmental/focal disease are 58 and 85%, respectively. Among all procedures, suction blister epidermal grafts and thin and ultra-thin split-thickness grafts seem to be the most effective procedures, with overall success rates of 80%. The least successful method was hair grafting, with an overall success rate of 50%. Among cellular grafts, all techniques seem to be equally effective with success rates of 61–64% for noncultured epidermal cell suspension, cultured melanocytes, and cultured epidermis. The success rates in bilateral vitiligo including generalized and acrofacial vitiligo were less than those in segmental or focal vitiligo with all the procedures. The success rates varied from 25% for hair grafting to 70% for thin and ultra-thin split-thickness grafts in bilateral vitiligo, while in segmental vitiligo, these ranged from 70% for hair grafting to 100% for thin and ultra-thin split-thickness skin grafts. The success rates in patients aged <20 years and ≥20 years were 82 and 58%, respectively. Among adverse reactions, hyperpigmentation in 32% and infection in 6% and contact dermatitis in 1% of the patients were observed.

Segmental vitiligo and piebaldism, responded in most cases with 100% repigmentation, regardless of the surgical method used.[18] For these types of vitiligo, surgery seems to be the method of choice. The ultra thin epidermal sheet method gives somewhat better overall results, but it is the method that gives the worst outcome in knee and elbow areas (mobility area). Irrespective of the method, fingers, palm and sole are the most difficult areas to repigment. The trunk and the arms and legs (not including elbows and knees) responded best. Patients with increasing and/or extensive vitiligo vulgaris more often showed incomplete repigmentation. They also had a lower chance of retaining their repigmentation compared with those with less extensive vitiligo. Patients in whom untreated white lesions had increased in recent years tended to respond less well to transplantation, compared with patients with unchanged or decreased lesions. Within the vitiligo vulgaris group, patients with short disease duration or with small total vitiligo area responded best to transplantation. The subgroup of vitiligo vulgaris patients with hypothyroidism tends to respond less well to transplantation and they were generally older at vitiligo onset. Slight hyperpigmentation is common, especially when ultra thin split thickness skin graft (STSG-UT) and blister epidermal split thickness skin

D. K. Gupta, *Microskin Grafting for Vitiligo*,
DOI: 10.1007/978-1-84882-605-2_20, © Springer Science + Business Media B.V. 2009

graft (STSG-BE) had been used. The color match is better in punch when compared to STSG-BE. In the recipient site, cobblestone appearance is the predominant complication in punch grafts whereas hyperpigmentation and thickening of grafts were common in STSG-BE. In the donor site, superficial scarring and hypopigmentation are the common findings in Punch skin graft, whereas hyperpigmentation is the main problem in STSG-BE. The results are significantly better in segmental/focal vitiligo than in the generalized type and in individuals <20 years of age.[19]

Autologous transplanted epidermal cell suspensions followed 3 weeks later by UV irradiation twice per week, for approximately 2 months, leads to repigmentation of at least 70% of the treated area in 55%, 57%, and 77% of the actively treated lesions 3, 6, and 12 months respectively, after treatment.[20]

The outcome of surgery is good in stable lesions whereas unstable lesions respond poorly. Thus, the stability status of vitiligo is the single, most important prerequisite in case selection. However, despite many studies, there is no consensus regarding the minimum required period of stability. The recommended period of stability in different studies has varied from 4 months to 3 years. Most authors have suggested that vitiligo can be classified as being stable, when there is no progression of old lesions and/or development of new lesions during the past 1 year. Segmental and nonsegmental vitiligo has been postulated to have a different etiopathogenesis and clinical course, by many investigators. Segmental vitiligo ceases to progress after a short period while nonsegmental vitiligo, thought to be of autoimmune origin, can progress continuously at a gradual rate throughout life.

As such, there are no uniformly acceptable measurement tools and indices for measurement of the efficacy of outcomes, of the surgical modalities of vitiligo treatment. Assessment of the quality of life and global assessment should be performed because the percentage of repimentation may not always be a good indicator of patient satisfaction. Patient's surgical outcome should be evaluated with holistic approach, which includes the extent of pigmentation, color match and complications of donor and recipient areas simultaneously. The excellent pigment recovery may be marred with hypertrophic scars, keloids and hyperpigmentation or patchy pigmentation.

20.1 Surgical Outcome and Benefits of Microskin Grafting

Apart from surgical contraindications, the stability status of vitiligo is the single, most important prerequisite in case selection. No patient must be operated if the vitiligo is unstable and progressive. Repigmentation obtained lasts long, as more than 95% of the patients have stayed pigmented. Considering the aesthetic outcome and the ability to treat larger area in a single sitting with very small skin, this technique may replace the present methods of surgical treatment of stable vitiligo, at practically no cost and no hi-tech laboratory and other infrastructure.

20.1.1 What Need to Be Followed in Microskin Grafting?

1. Select a patient with stable vitiligo (stable for last 6–12 months).I personally prefer a patient of more than 12 months stability.
2. Donor area to be selected from cosmetically insignificant site e.g. gluteal region, gluteal fold, anterolateral and posterior aspect of thigh and medial aspect of upper arm (Fig. 20.1).
3. Only harvest thin (0.2–0.3 mm) or ultra thin (0.08–0.15 mm) split thickness skin graft by using Silver's knife, Humby knife or any power dermatome. Using

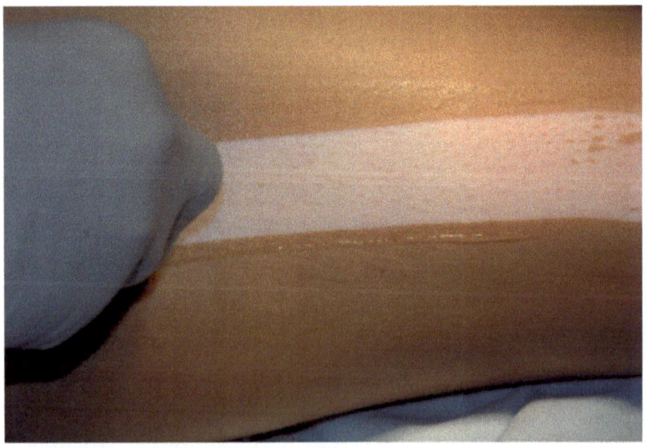

Fig. 20.1 Smooth and clean, thin or ultra thin graft harvesting from lateral aspect of thigh

thin or ultra thin grafts is the only way to avoid near total donor site deformities (Fig. 20.2a, b).

4. Skin graft should be transformed into microskin grafts (0.2–0.8 mm) by sharp scissors to minimize microskin graft damage.
5. Always use expansion method to cover maximum vitiliginous area by using small donor area. Commonly used donor to recipient area ratio varies from 1:5 to 1:15.
6. Uniform distributions of the MSGs are very well needed for uniform early pigmentation with excellent color match.

20.1.2 What are the Benefits of Microskin Grafting?

1. This procedure is safe, simple, easy to learn, cost effective and gives excellent results within 3–5 months time even in difficult to treat sites like lips, eyelids, nipples and areolas, elbows, knees and genitals. In areas like fingers, toes, palms and soles, more time is needed to achieve near total pigmentation.
2. This procedure gives good expansion ratio with fast pigmentation and good quality color match.
3. Practically no donor and recipient area deformity.
4. Simple office based procedure
5. No special laboratory and infra structure
6. More than 1,000 cm^2 vitiliginous area can be treated easily in one operative session in less than 2 hours time and at practically no cost. I routinely treat 2–1,500 cm^2 area of stable vitiligo in a patient in single session, with uniform pigmentation and excellent color match.
7. It is always preferable to treat all the vitiliginous lesions in a patient in one session rather than in multiple sessions after confirming the stability of the disease for at least 1 year.
8. This technique is also very useful in the management of leukotrichia. Hair pigmentation starts from 3 months onwards (Fig. 20.3).
9. This technique is again very good in pigmenting post burn leukoderma and dyschromia without the inherent side effects of split thickness skin sheet grafting.
10. Complete uniform pigmentation is based on donor to recipient area ratio. Acral areas like toes and fingers always take longer time than that of other areas.
11. *Microskin grafting is the best method to remove surgical stigma left behind, following punch grafting on donor and recipient areas.*

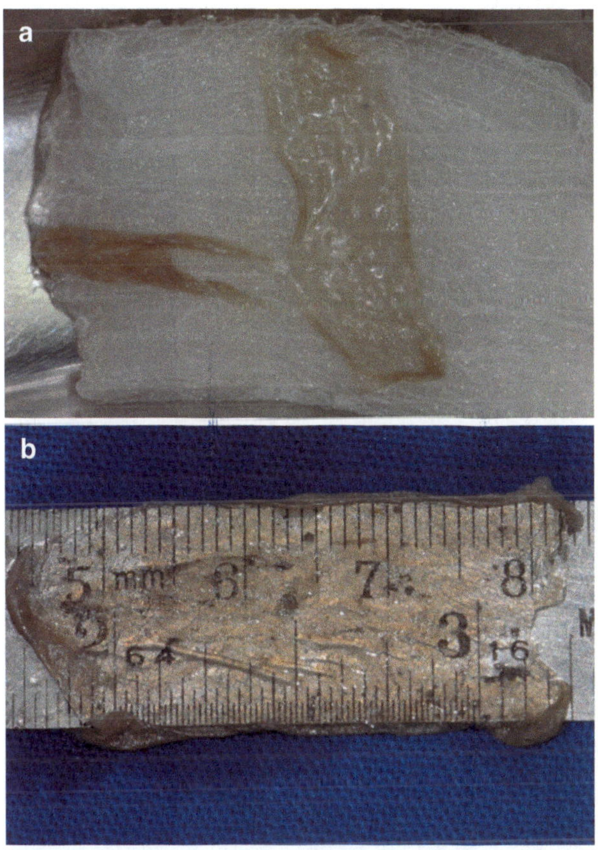

Fig. 20.2 (**a–b**) Ultra thin split thickness skin graft

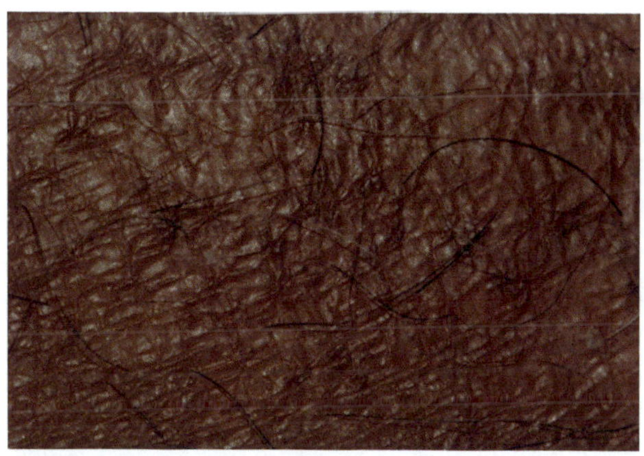

Fig. 20.3 Repigmentation of hairs in leukotrichia at 4 months. Implanted microskin grafts can also be seen

20.1.3 Donor to Recipient Area Expansion Ratio

- Complete pigmentation, except on acral areas, is achieved by direct spread of the MSGs by the spatula (donor-to-recipient expansion 1:1 ratio) in less than 3 months time. *Presently I stopped using this direct method due to better results obtained by floatation and spraying methods with utilization of very small donor areas.*
- Expansion ratio (donor-to-recipient expansion 1:3–1:4) – complete pigmentation in 3–4 months time (Fig. 20.4).
- Expansion ratio (donor-to-recipient expansion 1:5–1:10) – complete uniform pigmentation in 4–5 months time (Fig. 20.5a, b, 20.6a, b, 20.7a, b, 20.8).
- Expansion ratio (donor-to-recipient expansion 1:15) – complete pigmentation in 4–7 months time with good color match (Figs. 20.9).
- Expansion ratio (donor-to-recipient expansion >1:25) (Fig. 20.10)

20.1.4 Caution!

Expansion more than 1:15 may leave behind skip vitiliginous areas. I prefer donor to recipient area expansion from 1:5 to 1:15 for quick, complete and uniform pigment recovery in less than 6 months time. It is advised to keep donor-to-recipient expansion ratio not more than1:3–1:4 in acral, palmer, planter and lip

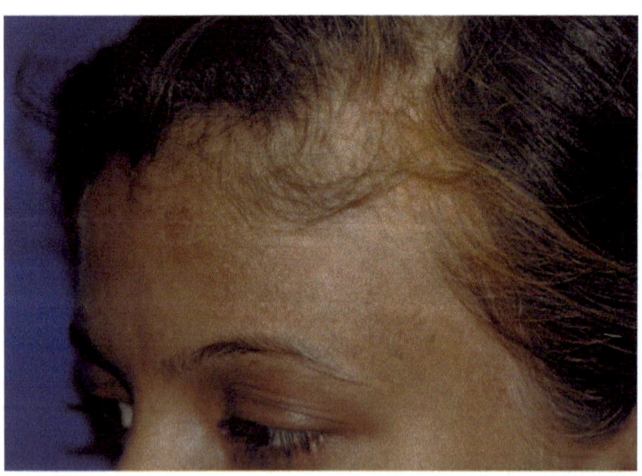

Fig. 20.4 Complete pigmentation at 3.5 months time with 1:4 expansion ratio

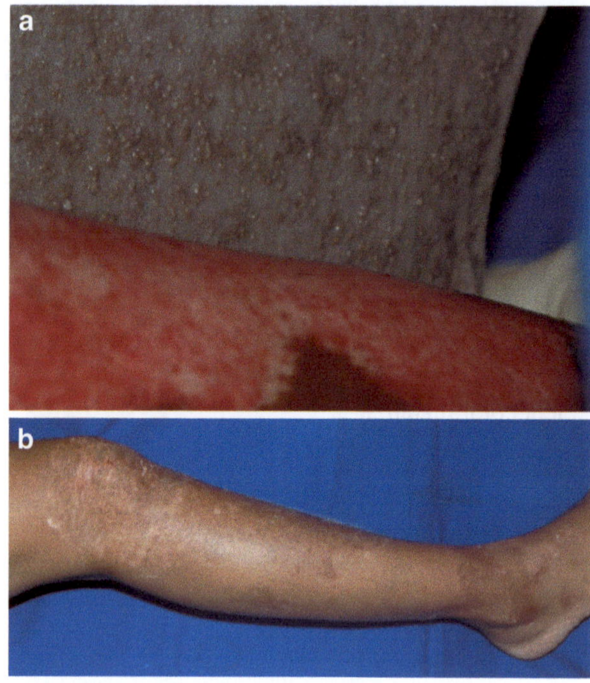

Fig. 20.5 (**a**) Donor to recipient area expansion ratio 1:5. (**b**) Pigmentation at 3.5 months

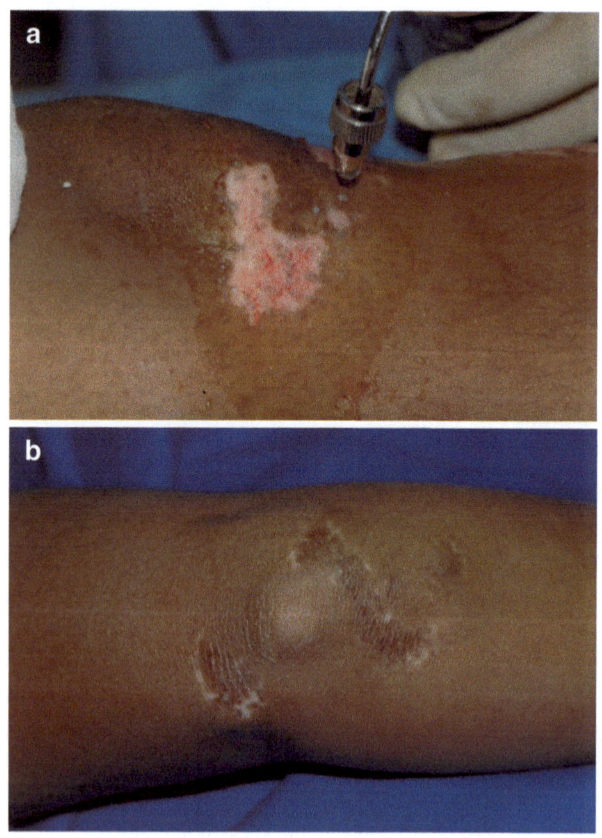

Fig. 20.6 (**a**) Donor to recipient area expansion ratio 1:8. (**b**) Pigmentation at 2.5 months time

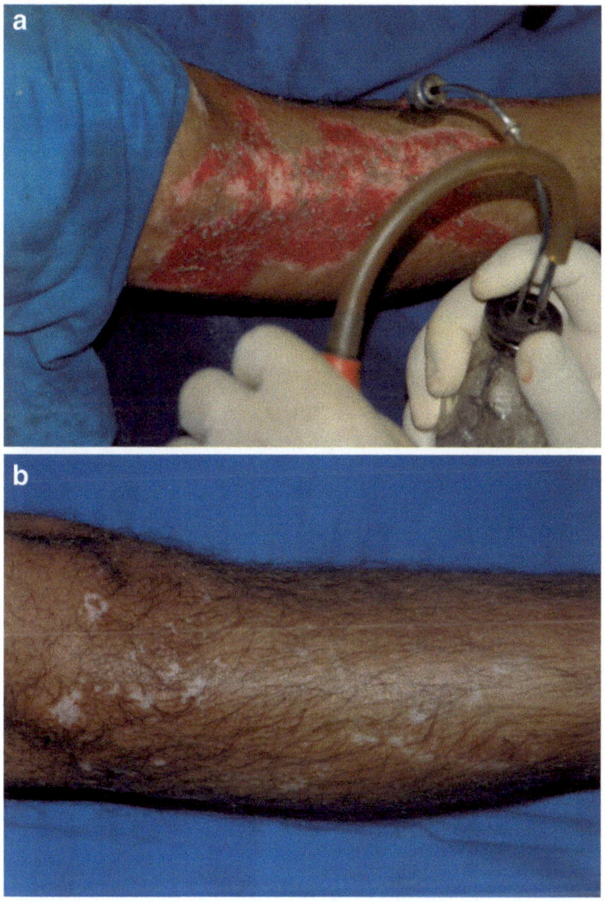

Fig. 20.7 (**a**) Donor to recipient area expansion ratio 1:8. (**b**) Pigmentation achieved at 3.5 months time

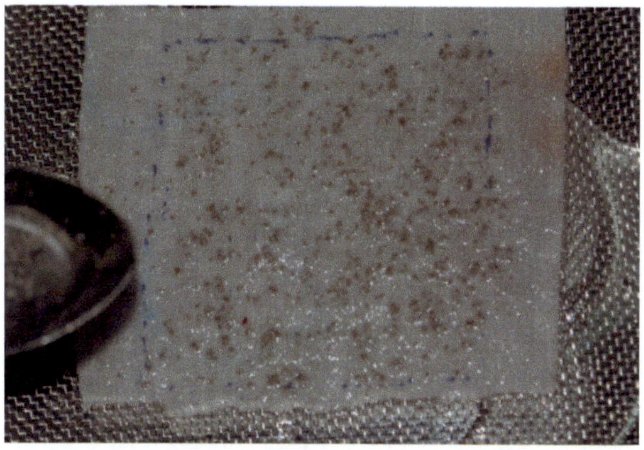

Fig. 20.8 Donor to recipient area expansion ratio 1:10. MSGs spread out over muslin cloth by floatation method

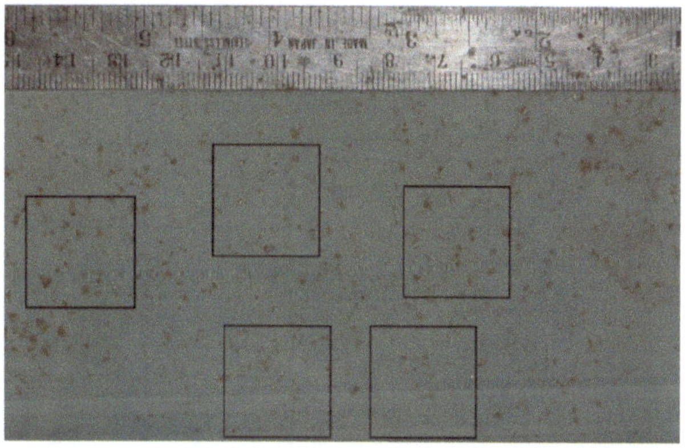

Fig. 20.10 Average donor to recipient area expansion ratio 1:25. MSGs spread out over muslin cloth by spraying method.

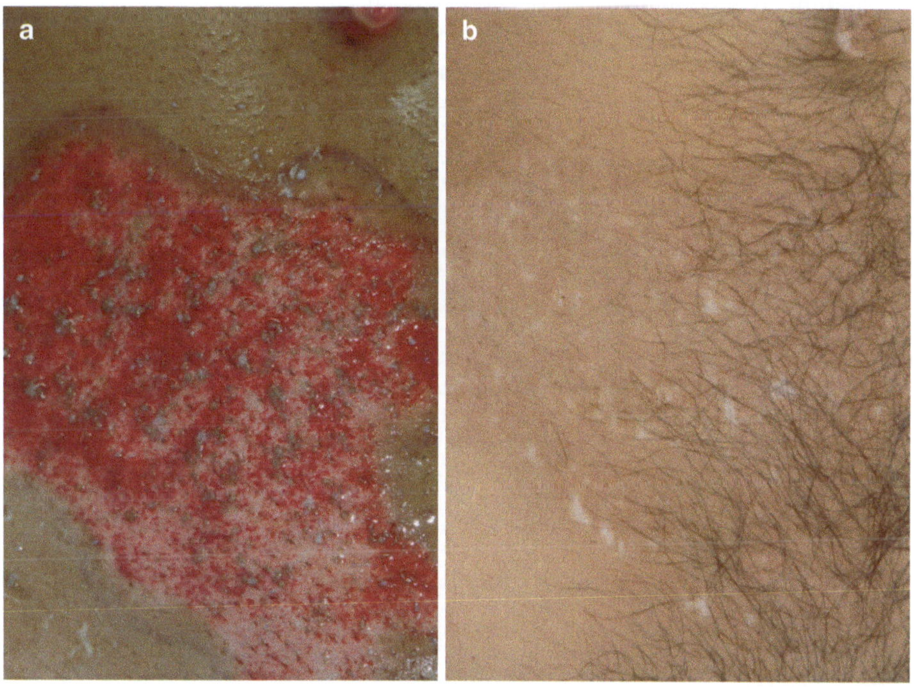

Fig. 20.9 (**a**) 1:15 expansion ratio. (**b**) Little less than complete pigmentation at 3.5 months time

vitiligo. If the extensive vitiligo becomes active during recovery of surgical treatment, then it should be controlled by systemic steroids or combination of systemic PUVA/PUVASOL and steroids. If the patient is already on systemic steroids, then it should not be stopped abruptly but continued till complete pigmentation is achieved and then gradually tapered down.

All stable generalized vitiligo patients should be kept on systemic PUVA or PUVASOL (psoralen + ultraviolet A therapy of solar origin) after microskin grafting to enhance pigment recovery. Segmental/focal stable vitiligo does not require any supporting medical therapy as above, but advised to expose treated area in sun for about 10–15 minutes daily.

In future, the method that gives a wider coverage in single operative session and in short operating time, with a less amount of donor tissue utilization and without any donor and recipient area complications, will succeed, if it is economical and easily available. This procedure of microskin grafting fulfils all the above requirements in treating stable, segmental and generalized vitiligo.

Microskin grafting will remain the mainstay of vitiligo surgical treatment by virtue of their simplicity, cost effectiveness, efficacy and ability to treat stable vast vitiliginous area in one session without leaving any donor and recipient area morbidity. This procedure of microskin grafting in treatment of vitiligo is certainly going to replace the punch grafting, hair follicular grafting, suction blister grafting and split thickness sheet skin grafting in the coming times. The results obtained even in 3–5 months time are much better than cellular grafts at practically no cost and time involvement.

References

1. Njoo MD, Westerhof W, Bos JD, Bossuyt MM. A systematic review of autologous transplantation methods in vitiligo. *Arch Dermatol.* 1998;134:1543–1545.
2. Guerra L, Capurro S, Melchi E. Treatment of "stable" vitiligo by timed surgery and transplantation of cultured epidermal autografts. *Arch Dermatol.* 2000;36:1380–1389.
3. Savant SS. Therapeutic spot and regional dermabrasion in stable vitiligo. *Indian J Dermatol Venereol Leprol.* 1996;62: 139–145.
4. Savant SS, Shenoy S. Chemical peeling with phenol for the treatment of stable vitiligo and alopecia areata. *Indian J Dermatol Venereol Leprol.* 1999;65:93–98.
5. Behl PN, Azad O, Kah R, Shrivastava G. Autologous thin Thiersch's grafts in vitiligo: experience of 8000 cases, 50,000 grafts (1959–1998) with modified technique in 198 cases in the year 1997–1998. *Indian J Dermatol Venereol Leprol.* 1999;65:117–121.
6. Savant SS. Autologous miniature punch grafting in stable vitiligo. *Indian J Dermatol Venereol Leprol.* 1992;58: 310–314.
7. Lontz W, Olsson MJ, Medllmann G, Lerner AB. Pigment cell transplantation for treatment of vitiligo: a progress report. *J Am Acad Dermatol.* 1994;30:591–597.
8. Kahn AM, Cohen MJ. Repigmentation in vitiligo patients. Melanocyte transfer via ultra thin grafts. *J Dermatol Surg.* 1998;24:365–367.
9. Chen YF, Yang PY, Hu DN. Treatment of vitiligo by transplantation of cultured pure melanocyte suspension. Analysis of 120 cases. *J Am Acad Dermatol.* 2004;51:68–74.
10. Mulekar SV. Melanocyte-keratinocyte cell transplantation: surgical therapy of vitiligo. *Int j Dermatol.* 2003;42: 132–136.
11. Mulekar SV. Long term follow-up study of segmental and focal vitiligo treated by autologous non cultured melanocytes-keratinocyte cell transplantation. *Arch Dermatol.* 2004;140: 1211–1215.
12. Savant SS. Vitiligo surgery: which? where? why? In: Savant SS ed. *Textbook of Dermatosurgery and Cosmetology*, 2nd edn. Mumbai: ASCAD; 2005:394–397.
13. Mutalik S, Ginzberg A. Surgical management of stable vitiligo: A review with personal experience. *J Dermatol Surg.* 2000;26:248–254.
14. Van Geel N, Ongenae K, Naeyaert JM. Surgical techniques for vitiligo: a review. *Dermatology.* 2001;202:162–166.
15. Yar M, Gilchrist B. Vitiligo. The evolution of cultured epidermal autografts and other surgical treatment modalities. *Arch Dermatol.* 2001;37:348–349.
16. Mahajan BB, Garg G, Gupta RR. Evaluation of cosmetic tattooing in localised stable vitiligo. *Int J Dermatol.* 2002;29: 726–730.
17. Gupta S, Kumar B. Epidermal grafting in vitiligo: influence of age, site of lesion and type of disease on outcome. *J Am Acad Dermatol.* 2003;49:99–104.
18. Olsson MJ, Juhlin L. *Br J Dermatol.* 2002;147(5):893–904.
19. Gupta S, Kumar B. *J Am Acad Dermatol.* 2003;49(1): 99–104.
20. van Geel N, Ongenae K, De Mil M, Haeghen YV, Vervaet C, Naeyaert JM. *Arch Dermatol.* 2004;140(10):1203–1208.

Appendix 1

Consent form for Vitiligo surgery

1. (name)-----------------, aged-------years, residing at (address)-------------------- have been advised to undergo surgery for my skin condition, Vitiligo.

I hereby give consent after being explained in a language that I understand about the procedure by Dr. --------------

1. I am aware that Vitiligo is a disease with a chronic, recurrent course.
2. I am aware that surgery is only a cosmetic procedure and other concomitant medical treatments may be essential. Surgery will not alter the course of the disease or prevent any recurrence. I am aware that the practice of medicine and surgery is not an exact science, and I acknowledge that no guarantees have been made to me as to the results of the operation or procedure.
3. My disease has been stable for the last-------months/year. I have no tendency for keloids.
4. I am aware that the exact course of the disease can not be predicted and, though the disease is stable at present, flare-ups and recurrences may occur at any time, in any part of the body.
5. I have been explained the procedure of the operation as follows:
   a) The procedure will be done under local anesthesia, under regional anaesthesia or under general anaesthesia. I recognize that when general anesthesia is used it presents additional risks over which the above doctors have no control, and I agree to discuss the risks of general anesthesia with the anesthesiologist before surgery is performed.
   b) The donor area is from thigh/gluteal area/gluteal fold/groin area/inner arm/axillary fold/post auricular area.
   c) The donor graft will be taken by grafting knife/dermatome.
   d) Recipient area will be abraded by dermabrader/laser/ultrasonic and then the graft applied, sealed by dressing.
6. I am aware that avoiding movements and taking care of the recipient area is essential for optimal results.
7. I am aware that I may experience some pain postoperatively and may need to take analgesics.

8. Donor area will need dressing; the donor area may take 2-3 weeks to heal.
9. I am aware that for optimal cosmetic results, it may take from six months to one year. I may need to take medical treatment during this period.
10. I am also aware that the grafted area may not match in texture and appearance with the surrounding skin. A perfect match with the surrounding normal skin may not always be possible.
11. I consent to be photographed before, during, and after the treatment; that these photographs shall be the property of the above doctors and may be published in scientific journals and/or shown for scientific reasons.
12. I agree to keep the above doctors informed of any change of address so that they can notify me of any late findings, and I agree to cooperate with the above doctors in my care after surgery until completely discharged.
13. I am not known to be allergic to anything except: (list)

I HAVE READ THE ABOVE CONSENT AND RECEIVED A COPY OF IT. I FULLY UNDERSTAND THE CONTENTS OF THE CONSENT AND AUTHORIZE AND REQUEST THE ABOVE DOCTORS TO PERFORM THIS SURGICAL PROCEDURE ON ME. THE CONSENT FORM HAS BEEN SIGNED BY ME WHEN I WAS NOT UNDER THE INFLUENCE OF ANY DRUGS.

Signature of the doctor

(Name ____________________________)

Date:Time

Signature of the Witness 1

(Name: ___________________________)

Date:Time

Signature of the patient

(Name: ______________________________)

Date:Time

Signature of witness 2

(Name: ______________________________)

Date:Time

IF PATIENT IS A MINOR, COMPLETE THE FOLLOWING:

Patient is a minor _________ years of age, and we, the under signed, are the parents, guardians, or legal representatives of the patient.

____

(Witness)

____

(Parent or legal guardian)

____

(Witness)

____

(Parent or legal guardian)

Index

MIX
Papier aus verantwortungsvollen Quellen
Paper from responsible sources
FSC® C105338

If you have any concerns about our products,
you can contact us on
ProductSafety@springernature.com

In case Publisher is established outside the EU,
the EU authorized representative is:
Springer Nature Customer Service Center GmbH
Europaplatz 3, 69115 Heidelberg, Germany

Printed by Libri Plureos GmbH
in Hamburg, Germany